Reconceiving Medical Ethics

Continuum Studies in Philosophy

Series Editor: James Fieser, University of Tennessee at Martin, USA

Continuum Studies in Philosophy is a major monograph series from Continuum. The series features first-class scholarly research monographs across the whole field of philosophy. Each work makes a major contribution to the field of philosophical research.

Aesthetic in Kant, James Kirwan

Analytic Philosophy: The History of an Illusion, Aaron Preston

Aquinas and the Ship of Theseus, Christopher Brown

Augustine and Roman Virtue, Brian Harding

The Challenge of Relativism, Patrick Phillips

Demands of Taste in Kant's Aesthetics, Brent Kalar

Descartes and the Metaphysics of Human Nature, Justin Skirry

Descartes' Theory of Ideas, David Clemenson

Dialectic of Romanticism, Peter Murphy and David Roberts

Duns Scotus and the Problem of Universals, Todd Bates

Hegel's Philosophy of Language, Jim Vernon

Hegel's Philosophy of Right, David James

Hegel's Theory of Recognition, Sybol S.C. Anderson

The History of Intentionality, Ryan Hickerson

Kantian Deeds, Henrik Jøker Bjerre

Kierkegaard, Metaphysics and Political Theory, Alison Assiter

Kierkegaard's Analysis of Radical Evil, David A. Roberts

Leibniz Re-interpreted, Lloyd Strickland

Metaphysics and the End of Philosophy, HO Mounce

Nietzsche and the Greeks, Dale Wilkerson

Origins of Analytic Philosophy, Delbert Reed

Philosophy of Miracles, David Corner

Platonism, Music and the Listener's Share, Christopher Norris

Popper's Theory of Science, Carlos Garcia

Postanalytic and Metacontinental, edited by James Williams, Jack Reynolds, James Chase and Ed Mares

Rationality and Feminist Philosophy, Deborah K. Heikes

Re-thinking the Cogito, Christopher Norris

Role of God in Spinoza's Metaphysics, Sherry Deveaux

Rousseau and Radical Democracy, Kevin Inston

Rousseau and the Ethics of Virtue, James Delaney

Rousseau's Theory of Freedom, Matthew Simpson

Spinoza and the Stoics, Firmin DeBrabander

Spinoza's Radical Cartesian Mind, Tammy Nyden-Bullock

St. Augustine and the Theory of Just War, John Mark Mattox

St. Augustine of Hippo, R. W. Dyson

Thomas Aquinas & John Duns Scotus, Alex Hall

Tolerance and the Ethical Life, Andrew Fiala

Reconceiving Medical Ethics

Edited by
Christopher Cowley

Continuum Studies in Philosophy

continuum

Continuum International Publishing Group

The Tower Building
11 York Road
London SE1 7NX

80 Maiden Lane
Suite 704
New York NY 10038

www.continuumbooks.com

British Library Cataloguing-in-Publication Data
A catalogue record for this book is available from the British Library.

ISBN: HB: 978-1-4411-2338-1

Library of Congress Cataloguing-in-Publication Data
Reconceiving medical ethics/edited by Christopher Cowley.
p. cm. – (Continuum studies in philosophy)
Includes bibliographical references and index.
ISBN 978-1-4411-2338-1 (hardcover: alk. paper) – ISBN 978-1-4411-2127-1 (ebook pdf : alk. paper) – ISBN 978-1-4411-0397-0 (ebook epub : alk. paper) 1. Medical ethics. I. Cowley, Christopher, 1967- II. Title. III. Series.
R724.R426 2012
174.2–dc23 2011031713

Typeset by Deanta Global Publishing Services, Chennai, India
Printed and bound in Great Britain

Contents

Contributors

Nafsika Athanassoulis has held posts as Lecturer in Ethics at Keele University and Lecturer in Philosophy at the University of Leeds. She is the author of *Morality, Moral Luck and Responsibility* (Palgrave 2005) and editor of *Philosophical Reflections on Medical Ethics* (Palgrave 2005) and with Samantha Vice, of *The Moral Life: essays in honour of John Cottingham* (Palgrave 2008). Her research interests include Aristotle and virtue ethics, medical ethics, moral education and the philosophy of risk (on the latter she has published extensively in collaboration with Allison Ross), and she is currently working on a textbook on virtue ethics for Continuum Press.

Alastair V. Campbell is the Chen Su Lan Centennial Professor of Medical Ethics and the Director of the Centre for Biomedical Ethics in the Yong Loo Lin School of Medicine of the National University of Singapore. Previously, he was Professor of Biomedical Ethics, University of Otago and then Professor of Ethics in Medicine, University of Bristol. He is a former President of the International Association of Bioethics. His recent books include *Health as Liberation* (1996), *Medical Ethics* (with D.G. Jones and G. Gillet, 3rd Edition 2005) and *The Body in Bioethics* (2009). He was formerly chair of the Ethics and Governance Council of UK Biobank and Vice-Chair of the UK Retained Organs Commission. Professor Campbell is currently a member of the Bioethics Advisory Committee to the Singapore Government. He was recently elected a Fellow of the Royal Society of Edinburgh.

Christopher Cowley is a lecturer at the School of Philosophy of University College, Dublin. He works in moral philosophy, moral psychology and applied ethics. He is the author of *Medical Ethics: Ordinary Concepts, Ordinary Lives* (Palgrave 2008), and is currently writing a monograph on the philosophy of autobiography.

Gaëlle Fiasse is Associate Professor at McGill University in the Department of Philosophy (Faculty of Arts) and in the Faculty of Religious Studies. Fiasse specializes in the history of philosophy and ethics, and in particular in Aristotle and Paul Ricœur. Her current research concerns the question of forgiveness and the theme of fragility. She was awarded a grant from the *Fonds québécois de la recherche sur la société et la culture* (FQRSC) for her project on forgiveness and another grant from the Social Sciences and Humanities Research Council of Canada (SSHRC) for her research on fragility. In addition to articles in French and English for journals and books, Fiasse has published *L'autre et l'amitié chez Aristote et Paul Ricœur. Analyses éthiques et ontologiques*, Louvain: Peeters 2006; and *Paul Ricœur. De l'homme faillible à l'homme capable*. Paris: Presses Universitaires de France 2008.

Julian C. Hughes is a Consultant in Old Age Psychiatry in Northumbria Healthcare NHS Foundation Trust and an Honorary Professor of Philosophy of Ageing at the Institute for Ageing and Health, Newcastle University, UK. He has studied Philosophy at both undergraduate and postgraduate levels. His writings and research focus on philosophical and ethical issues raised in connection with ageing and dementia. Edited, co-edited or co-authored books include: *Dementia: Mind, Meaning, and the Person* (Oxford University Press 2006), *Palliative Care in Severe Dementia* (Quay Books 2006), *Ethical Issues in Dementia Care: Making Difficult Decisions* (Jessica Kingsley 2006), *Supportive Care for the Person with Dementia* (Oxford University Press 2010). In February 2011, his book, *Thinking Through Dementia* (Oxford University Press), was published. *Alzheimer's and Other Dementias: The Facts* was also published by Oxford University Press in September 2011.

Richard Huxtable is Reader in Medical Ethics & Law and the Deputy Director of the Centre for Ethics in Medicine at the University of Bristol. He has qualifications in Law (LLB (Hons.), Nottingham) and in socio-legal studies (MA, Sheffield), as well as a PhD in Law and Ethics in Medicine (Bristol). His academic work focuses primarily upon end-of-life decision-making and surgical ethics, and he has published widely in medical, legal and bioethical journals, in addition to authoring the books *Euthanasia, Ethics and the Law: From Conflict to Compromise* (Routledge-Cavendish 2007) and (with Dickenson & Parker) *The Cambridge Medical Ethics Workbook* (CUP 2nd ed. 2010). A long-standing participant in clinical ethics consultation, Huxtable works with the National Council for Palliative Care and the Bristol Clinical Ethics Advisory Group, having previously served on the Bath RUH Clinical Ethics Committee.

Rien Janssens graduated in theology at the Radboud University of Nijmegen in 1996. After graduation he did extensive international research on concepts and ethics of palliative care. He earned his doctorate degree in 2001. In 2004, he was appointed Assistant Professor of Medical Ethics at the VU Medical Centre in Amsterdam. His research interests include end-of-life care, medical decision-making at the end of life and research ethics.

David Albert Jones is Director of the Anscombe Bioethics Centre, Research Fellow in Bioethics at Blackfriars Hall, Oxford, and Visiting Professor at the Centre for Bioethics and Emerging Technologies, at St Mary's University College, Twickenham. Jones read Natural Sciences and Philosophy at Cambridge (1984-1987), and Theology at Oxford (1992-2000). His publications include *The Soul of the Embryo* (2004 Continuum), *Approaching the End* (2007 Oxford University Press) and *Angels: A History* (2010 Oxford University Press). Jones is on the national reference group of the Liverpool Care Pathway and was on a working party of the General Medical Council which helped draft its 2010 guidance on treatment and care towards the end of life.

D. K. Levy teaches at the University of Edinburgh in the department of philosophy, where he teaches moral philosophy and the history of philosophy. His published books and articles have concerned moral philosophy, Wittgenstein, and cognitive psychology. His research is oriented around understanding, especially moral understanding.

Eric Matthews is Emeritus Professor of Philosophy and Honorary Research Professor of Medical and Psychiatric Ethics at the University of Aberdeen. His main research interests are in Biomedical Ethics, the Philosophical Foundations of Psychiatry, and twentieth-century French philosophy, especially Maurice Merleau-Ponty. He has published many articles and some books in all these areas. His books include: *Rationing Medical Care on the Basis of Age: the moral dimensions* (with Elizabeth Russell), (Oxford and Seattle, Radcliffe Publishing, for the Nuffield Trust 2005); *Merleau-Ponty: A Guide for the Perplexed* (London and New York, Continuum 2006); and *Body-Subjects and Disordered Minds* (Oxford and New York, Oxford University Press 2007).

Cliona McGovern is a lecturer in Forensic & Legal Medicine in University College Dublin (UCD). She has a PhD in coroners' law and death investigation from the University of Sheffield and an MA in the medico-ethical aspects of the diagnosis of brain death from UCD. She was a member of the Working

Group on the Review of the Coroner Service with the Irish Government's Department of Justice, Equality and Law Reform. She compiled the draft rules for coroners, including best practice notes for post-mortem and retention of organs. She has also produced a report for the Department of Transport on single vehicle crashes and has published internationally on suicide in Ireland. She is a member of the Irish College of General Practitioners Research Ethics Committee, which reviews potential clinical trials in Ireland. She was the deputy editor for the Medico-Legal Journal of Ireland. In UCD, she lectures on aspects of forensic and legal medical to undergraduate medical, radiography and physiotherapy students and she lectures the graduate courses in Healthcare Risk Management & Quality and in Forensic Medicine.

Steve Ramplin is a consultant forensic psychiatrist based at Roseberry Park, Middlesbrough. He graduated from Newcastle university in 1995 and spent time outside medicine before training in psychiatry. He has a keen interest in philosophy and is studying for a Masters in Philosophy of Mental Health at the University of Central Lancashire. Exploring a fascination for the interplay between criminality and the mind, he has written about the medicalization of psychopathy, the phenomenology of paedophilia, homicidal somnambulism and whether Values-Based Medicine can provide an ethical framework for forensic psychiatry. His dissertation on the murder defence of diminished responsibility explores themes of moral responsibility and agency. He has also studied service-user perspectives and values within secure psychiatric settings.

Allison Ross is an independent scholar. She has taught philosophy at Roehampton University and professional ethics at the Centre for Professional Ethics at Keele University. Her research interests include various topics within what can broadly be called virtue ethics. In particular, she is interested in the development and deformation of character and in the role played by practical rationality in good moral decision-making. She has recently been working with Nafsika Athanassoulis on a series of papers which aim to develop a virtue ethics approach to the moral assessment of risk-taking.

Ruth Stirton is a Lecturer in Law at the University of Sheffield. She is a medical lawyer and bioethicist, whose main research interest is the ethical and legal implications of the use of predictive genetic information by third parties, such as insurers. She is currently working on a monograph exploring the legal rights that individuals have in relation to information about their genetic makeup. Her existing publications, as Ruth Wilkinson, include work on genetic discrimination, genetic exceptionalism in legislation and research ethics.

Mark Wicclair is Professor of Philosophy and Adjunct Professor of Community Medicine at West Virginia University and Adjunct Professor of Medicine at the University of Pittsburgh Center for Bioethics and Health Law. His primary areas of specialization are bioethics and applied ethics. His publications include articles and book chapters on conscientious objection in medicine, nursing, and pharmacy; futility; managed care; decision-making capacity; end-of-life decision-making; the ethics of decision-making in critical care; research and training with the dead; the obligations of adult children to frail elderly parents; pornography; and prostitution. He also has written an article and a book chapter on the television series, *House M.D.* He is the author of *Ethics and the Elderly* (Oxford University Press 1993) and *Conscientious Objection in Health Care: An Ethical Analysis* (Cambridge University Press 2011).

Guy Widdershoven is Professor of Philosophy and Ethics of Medicine, Head of the Department of Medical Humanities and senior researcher at the EMGO Institute for Health and Care Research of VU University Medical Center, Amsterdam. He has published on hermeneutic ethics and its application in empirical ethics, moral deliberation and ethics of chronic care (psychiatry and elderly care). His research topics include autonomy in chronic care, coercion in psychiatry, evaluation of moral deliberation projects, end-of-life issues, genetics and public health genomics. He is scientific director of the Netherlands School of Primary Care Research (CaRe) and president of the European Association of Centers of Medical Ethics (EACME).

Kristin Zeiler is Associate Professor in Ethics with a special focus on medical ethics at the Department of Medical and Health Sciences, Linköping University, Sweden. Her research focuses on ethical and philosophical issues arising within medicine and includes work in areas such as phenomenology of the body, medical ethics, global ethics and feminist theory. See Zeiler K. (2010) 'A Phenomenological Analysis of Bodily Self-awareness in Pain and Pleasure. On Bodily Dys-appearance and Eu-appearance' in: *Medicine, Health Care and Philosophy* vol. 13(4), pp. 333–342; Malmqvist E. and Zeiler K. (2010) 'Cultural Norms, the Phenomenology of Incorporation and the Experience of Having a Child Born with Ambiguous Sex' in: *Social Theory and Practice* vol. 36(1), pp. 157–164; and Zeiler K. (2009) 'Deadly pluralism? Why death concept, death definition, death criterion and death test pluralism should be allowed, even though it evokes some problems' in: *Bioethics* vol. 23, pp. 450–459

Introduction

Christopher Cowley

This anthology comprises a modest challenge, sometimes direct, sometimes implicit, to the mainstream Anglo-American conception of the discipline of medical ethics. It does so not by trying to fill the gaps with exotic topics of minority interest, but by re-examining some of the fundamental assumptions of the familiar philosophical arguments, and some of the basic situations (including the *descriptions* of the situations) that generate the issues.

The most important of such situations is the encounter between the doctor and the suffering patient. Before asking the mainstream question 'what are the doctor's obligations to the patient?', we believe that there are more important questions to ask first, such as: 'what is suffering, exactly, and how does it generate moral claims?', 'How does the suffering affect the patient's understanding of her own life?', 'How does the suffering enter into the relationship between patient and doctor?', 'What does the patient expect from the doctor, and when are such expectations legitimate?', 'What does the doctor need to do in order to understand the patient appropriately?', 'What exactly gives the doctor the right to touch the patient, to insert a needle into her?', 'What is the doctor's appropriate place in society?', 'How do doctors understand the prohibitions placed on them by their own profession and by the law?' Many of these questions will already have clear answers in non-philosophical terms, e.g. in terms of physiology, of psychology, of convention. Many of these questions will also strike mainstream philosophers as being trivial. It might seem obvious, for example, that medicine is a service like any other: the customer brings his defective property to the expert for repair, and it is the customer's free and informed consent that justifies the entire transaction. Several of the contributors challenge the view of medicine as a service, the view of the body as property, the view of consent as providing ultimate justification, and the view of the encounter as isolated from the rest of the patient's and doctor's lives.

In trying to answer these questions, some of the contributors will be making use of the work of philosophers often described as Continental or European. This will be a secondary purpose of the anthology: to reveal the relevance of Husserl, Heidegger, Merleau-Ponty, Foucault and Ricoeur in reconceiving the central problems that characterize the discipline of medical ethics. It is interesting that none of these authors were mentioned at all in the two major reference works that appeared in the last five years: Steinbock's *Oxford Handbook of Bioethics* (2009) and Singer and Viens's *Cambridge Textbook of Bioethics* (2008). Indeed, it is rare for any of these philosophers to make more than a token appearance on the curricula of the Anglo-American philosophy department. And yet these philosophers have advanced sophisticated ideas about embodiment, power, narrative, self-understanding and other-understanding.

With the above in mind, it is worth spelling out what we will *not* be doing in this volume. Most mainstream anthologies in bioethics or medical ethics are compilations of "–isms" and "issues". The first section might have a series of ethical theories such as utilitarianism and key concepts such as justice. The second section then collects together the big journalistic topics such as abortion and euthanasia and lays them out with arguments for and against. There is nothing wrong with this approach, but the existence of the *Oxford Handbook* and *the Cambridge Textbook* has obviated the need for another such volume, at least for the next few years. So this anthology is not aiming to provide a broad mainstream introduction to the discipline; it is written for a general reader already familiar with most of the –isms and the issues, most of the big newspaper debates and government policy disagreements. Nor does this anthology aim to provide the 'latest developments' in the mainstream fields, even if some of the authors will survey some of the latest developments in their own approaches.

Second, this is a book of *medical* ethics, which means that it is narrower than bioethics and omits topics such as animals, the environment, and research ethics. It also means that it is narrower than 'healthcare ethics' in that it is not primarily concerned with other healthcare professionals (nurses, physiotherapists, psychologists, social workers or hospital managers) – although many of the conclusions could be adapted without much loss to other professions.

Third, since we are focusing more on the ordinary encounter between doctor and patient, we will be avoiding some of the favourite topics of mainstream medical ethics, that is, those that comprise very abstract ideas or those that arise from very rare situations. This means that, with a couple of exceptions, we will not be discussing the following in any detail: resource allocation at the national or international level; the dilemmas brought forth by advanced technological developments such as stem cells, pre-implantation genetic diagnosis, or xenotransplantation; the abstractions and applications of ethical theories or of the Four-Principle accounts made famous by Beauchamp and Childress (2009).

Fourth, we will be restricting our discussions to modern Western societies, and especially those with a national health service such as in the UK and in most of Europe. Some points of comparison will also be made with the American context where relevant.

Summaries of the Contributions

Part I. The suffering patient, the suffering body.

We begin with the simple human experience of suffering, and more particularly of suffering localized within a part of one's body. The person is aware that something is wrong and this is the reason to go and see the doctor. But in order for the person to understand what it means to suffer from a broken leg or a chesty cough or chronic abdominal pain, we first need to understand what it means for one's experience of the world to be essentially embodied and for those experiences themselves to be situated within an on-going life. Sometimes in stark contrast to the person's own conception of her body and of her suffering body is the scientific or mechanistic model of understanding: the body as governed by myriad interconnected causal processes, more or less known, more or less predictable; the body as very much part of the natural world. Some of these processes contribute to healthy function, others inhibit it, and the doctor-scientist wields a variety of tools to diagnose and treat as best she can.

Alastair Campbell opens with a discussion of the 2001 Alder Hey scandal in Britain, when it was revealed that organs of dead children had been routinely removed and retained by the Alder Hey hospital pathologists over many years without informing the children's parents. According to one popular conception of the body in philosophy and in medicine, the body is just a machine, and so the dead body is a useless abandoned machine: the Alder Hey parents' furious reaction is therefore at best incomprehensible, at worst, selfish for hindering scientific progress. Indeed, Campbell cites philosopher John Harris's bewilderment. However, what Harris fails to understand, according to Campbell, are the *meanings* which the human bodies, living and dead, possess in human lives. We cannot simply ignore or abandon these meanings by declaring the body to be no more than a vehicle for transporting persons around. At the same time, to understand the body as meaningful is not to deny the reality of death: a husband kissing the brow of his dead wife is expressing his love, in a completely natural way, even if he does not expect her to acknowledge his kiss (p. 17). Campbell then considers the degree to which one's body, one's blood and one's internal organs can plausibly and coherently be considered as one's property. The concept of property involves a range of implications, and one's ethical views of the treatment of dead bodies and their organs, as well as the full meaning of any donation or organs or bodies, will depend on which of these implications are seen as most relevant.

Paul Ricœur is justly famous for his work on interpretation and narrative, some of which has found its way into medical ethics through the recent interest in the narrative aspect of illness and suffering (for example, Brody 2002). However, Gaëlle Fiasse explores other crucial aspects of Ricœur's ethics and his work specifically on medicine, above all his emphasis on the encounter between physician and patient. His analysis of this relationship helps to ground an ethics that precedes the norms and duties characteristic of the Kantian mainstream. Even though norms and precepts should be taken into consideration, argues Ricœur, they presuppose the face-to-face relationship, as well as the Golden Rule and the use of Aristotelian practical wisdom. In every 'pact of care' (*pacte de soins*), different aspects of solicitude are at stake in spite of the asymmetry between the medical worker and the suffering patient; and only by properly *attending* to the other can this asymmetry be somewhat corrected. This attention involves the physician's attempt, by a more faithful 'translation' of the patient's words, to better understand the specific nature of the patient's fragility, as well as the nature of the physician's own fragility. Such translation is an integral part of the proper mode of being with that other.

While normative moral theory has developed into a stable set of debates between consequentialism, deontology and virtue ethics, the third has only been applied to medical ethics by a handful of philosophers, some of them cited by Kristin Zeiler in her contribution. The advantage of virtue ethics approaches is that they can take into account the character of the doctor and its development – for better or for worse – through medical school and subsequent professional life. It is all very well discussing the right or best thing to do in a given situation, but if the doctor can't perceive it, cannot deliberate about it properly, and does not feel the appropriate emotions in response, then she may be unable to choose that action. In her contribution, Zeiler takes this virtue ethics work further by applying it in conjunction with Merleau-Ponty's phenomenology of bodily skill development. For Zeiler claims that there is a bodily dimension to ethical learning as well, and that the acquisition of virtues-as-skills can have a direct effect on perceptual and emotional engagement.

Part II. When high-tech medicine fails: old age, dying and mental illness

Medical ethics tends to share the prejudice of television medical drama: there is a lot of attention to high technology and to high-stress life-and-death decisions. And yet both ignore the huge number of patients with much less glamorous ailments. First, medical ethics tends to ignore the ordinary slow business of growing old. Part of growing old, of course, is to suffer a stroke or a cardiac arrest, but most of it involves a tediously gradual decline in function, and a slow increase in dependency that is usually managed by occupational therapists and social workers rather than doctors. By far the main problems with old age are not medical but social and spiritual. However, when doctors do intervene, the temptation is to fix the mechanical problem and then send the patient away, rather than seeing the intervention as an integral part of a wider, imperfect attempt by society to meet the needs of the increasing numbers of elderly. With a few notable exceptions, noted by Eric Matthews in his piece, medical ethics also tends to ignore the elderly other than as contingent bearers of interesting conditions.

One essential aspect of old age is dependency. But as Matthews explains, this dependency comprises more than a mere loss of skill and function (mirroring the accumulation of skill and function in childhood and adolescence): for the loss is exacerbated by the responses of others, who will sometimes talk down to the elderly in the same way as they talk down to children. It might seem that the solution to this tendency is to reaffirm the importance of individual autonomy. However, this is often problematic with the elderly because their autonomy seems compromised by their increasing dependence, and, in the case of dementia, by their loss of continuity with their earlier self. Using the work of George Agich and Maurice Merleau-Ponty, Matthews proceeds to re-examine the concept of autonomy in order to suggest a dialogical rather than confrontational model, where such dialogue can accommodate dependency, and open greater possibilities for the young – including young doctors and carers – to understand the old.

If the lack of attention in medical ethics to the ordinary business of ageing is surprising, given the fact that the vast majority of us will grow old, then the lack of attention to the ordinary business of dying is even more surprising. By dying, I mean the terminal phase of life where scientific medicine can do no more except provide pain relief. Once again it is tempting to think that since medicine has given up, so too should medical ethics: all the difficult ethical decisions have been made. But palliative care and hospice care are nevertheless important parts of life precisely because this is a time when patients can organize and reflect on their lives. This is not just a matter of enjoying the good memories, tidying up one's affairs, and saying one's goodbyes: more importantly, it is a matter of making sense of one's life from a more objective, detached perspective. Finally, a discussion of palliative care is crucially important for medical ethics since it is the main alternative to euthanasia. Too often the euthanasia debate – perhaps the largest and most complicated debate in medical ethics – assumes that it is a matter of permitting or prohibiting in response to the patient's competent request. But too often that request is made in fear of a slow and undignified decline with poor palliative efforts, and those who would prohibit euthanasia might not sufficiently acknowledge their responsibility to make the alternative more palatable.

Rien Janssens and Guy Widdershoven provide an overview of the history of palliative and hospice care in the past half century, together with some of the justifications for it in the face of surprising social and medical resistance. Part of the problem with its acceptance and funding, they argue, have been some conceptual tensions and ambiguities. One such ambiguity is the place of death in discussions with the patient: how openly should the doctor or hospice worker mention it, especially when the patient is afraid? As in Matthews's piece, another ambiguity surrounds the concept of autonomy, and Janssens and Widdershoven outline some principles of 'hermeneutic ethics' (p. 79) to better characterize the nature of the relationship between doctor and patient, and the relationship between moral philosophy and the hospice situation. The most important principle of hermeneutic ethics is that the theoretical impetus has to be tempered by particular knowledge of the situation and by the understandings that the practitioners themselves have of the situation.

The ordinary business of ageing and dying is the most common example of the failure of high-tech medicine. Another is mental health, and the third and fourth chapters are about this. The first thing to realize is that a lot of mental illness is also pretty ordinary: low-grade depression and age-related senility are hardly rare. The second thing is that only a small portion of it is treatable by the standard tools of medicine, and such treatments are often pretty clumsy, merely controlling the symptoms rather than curing. Most mental illness involves suffering that is very different in kind from somatic suffering. As Steve Ramplin and Julian Hughes put it, there is something 'shocking' about mental illness (p. 84), perhaps because at a deeper level it undermines our own confidence in our grip on reality. This means that mental illness has the ability to 'change the conversation' in medical ethics, as they put it. To explore the difference between mental and somatic illness and the impact on medical ethics, they invoke two notions. The first is the Heideggerian notion of 'being-with-others' (together with the specific type of caring involved in such being, 'solicitude'). The second is the theory of 'values-based medicine' (VBM), most comprehensively developed by K. W. M. Fulford (2004). One of the reasons that mental illness poses such a challenge to medicine, argue Ramplin and Hughes, is precisely because it seems to undermine the value structures normally shared by patient and doctor.

Cowley considers the famous 1991 Dutch *Chabot* case, in which a somatically healthy 50-year-old woman, Mrs. Bosscher, asked psychiatrist Dr. Chabot to assist her to commit suicide. Dutch legislation permits physician-assisted suicide (PAS) and voluntary euthanasia in the event of 'unbearable and hopeless suffering'; the vast majority of requests come from competent patients with advanced cancer. Mrs. Bosscher claimed to be unbearably and hopelessly depressed after a bad marriage to an abusive alcoholic and after the deaths of both her sons (the first from suicide); Dr. Chabot believed her, and helped her to die, and his decision was essentially upheld by the Dutch Supreme Court. For the purposes of the article, Cowley accepts the legality of PAS as a response to somatic suffering, and accepts that Mrs. Bosscher's depression was 'justified' (to use George Graham's (1990) term), but argues that such mental suffering was of such a different kind that it could not justify suicide under Dutch procedures. This is because of the difficulty of demonstrating genuine hopelessness without corroboration from general disease statistics: every depression is unique in a way that every cancer is not, and so there is no way to predict the future course of a particular depression.

Part III. Autonomy and autonomous decision-making

The four chapters in this part pick up on the preceding discussions of autonomy. If there is one part of the ethics of medical practice that has changed enormously in the past half century, it is the attitude of the profession to patient consent. As a corrective to the paternalistic tendencies of those with excess power and knowledge, this is of course to be welcomed. However, there are still outstanding philosophical questions to ask about the nature of the patient's consent. Again, it is too simplistic to understand patient consent along the lines of the customer's consent to a service such as dry cleaning, not only because there are very few services that are as intrusive and dangerous as medicine, not only because the medical 'customer' often has so little idea of what medicine does and of what impact it will have on her, but mainly because there are few services which are the subject of such urgent and genuine need.

D. K. Levy begins this part by using the issue of autonomy to illuminate a facet in the disagreement between two views in ethical theory, consequentialist and deontologist. Roughly, consequentialists assess moral judgements about actions based on those actions' consequences, while deontologists assess those judgements with reference to duty. For example, judgements about medical treatments can be assessed, ranked, regarded as impermissible, etc. using the differing considerations central to these viewpoints. A commonplace of contemporary medical ethics is that considerations of autonomy must also weigh in the assessment of medical treatments. Levy argues that considerations of autonomy *cannot* be considered within the consequentialist viewpoint.Therefore, if autonomy is central to medical ethics, the presumption must be against assessing treatments from a consequentialist perspective. This conclusion is defended notwithstanding Levy's acknowledgement that there is a seemingly natural fit between medical ethics and consequentialism because of how consequentialism conceives all ethical challenges as practical problems. Certainly, consequentialism is well-suited to some practical problems, especially collective problems like allocating scarce resources. However, with individual patients, consequentialism is unable to take account of a patient's autonomous perspective. It must regard a patient as a constituent of a state of affairs, as the locus of contingent future welfare, which welfare is marshalled or conserved with indifference to who does the marshalling or conserving. The consequentialist viewpoint of an individual thereby precludes forms of attention – like pity or respect – that are intrinsically related to perceiving another's autonomy. In some cases, mercy, writes Levy, may even require a doctor to 'act contrary to what is indicated, e.g. by the patient's stated desire or by clinical best practice' (p. 115). Examples like mercy also show that there will be limits to the weight medical ethics should give to autonomy.

In the same way that medical ethics has often accorded only a grudging customer-service respect of patient autonomy, it has also accorded reluctant respect to autonomous wishes and refusals based on the patient's religious convictions. It is too easy for a doctor to say: 'human bodies are human bodies, religion has nothing to do with it'; just as it is too easy for a doctor to summon the hospital chaplain when the discussion becomes too spiritual for her liking. Surely the doctor has herself reflected on the big questions of life and death, even without the specific idiom of a religious doctrine and cosmology, and in that respect is perfectly qualified to engage with the patient's religious and spiritual concerns. This question should be distinguished from two others; first, from the striking but relatively rare cases such as the competent adult Jehovah's Witnesses legally refusing blood transfusions, knowing that their earthly life will end.[1] Second, it should be distinguished from the contributions to the *Cambridge Textbook* such as 'Hindu approaches to bioethics', which summarize specific *doctrinal* approaches to ethical questions separately, from a secular perspective. Instead, it is always worth bearing in mind how much so-called secular perspectives are often suffused with religious notions. Even the very idea of 'healing' is importantly ambiguous in this sense.

David Albert Jones begins his discussion of these questions by examining the claims of the Secular Medical Forum, who explicitly attempt to reduce the allegedly pernicious influence of religion on the optimal practice of scientific medicine. Such opposition is nothing new, as Jones traces its historical roots back at least 200 years. One reaction to this secular assault has been to argue that religion can do no harm and might actually benefit the suffering patient – but this, writes Jones, would be to misconstrue the place that religious beliefs have in people's lives. Indeed, 'Christianity may require actions that are a burden to mental health and which may have an adverse effect on the believer's subjective experience of well-being' (p. 140).

The third and fourth chapters in this part deal with the question of patient autonomy and consent indirectly, by examining the importance of the patient's particular understanding and appreciation of risks, and especially the risks posed by genetic illness. It is one thing to present a risk in terms of an inductive generalization of similar cases in the past: it is another for the patient to decide that something is too risky for her to undertake. Nafsika Athanassoulis and Allison Ross discuss (p. 149) the example of 60-year-old Thanos, who is diagnosed with stage 2 prostate cancer. Surgery offers the possibility of a cure, but also the risk of incontinence and erectile dysfunction. Although the likely progress of the cancer can be statistically predicted based on past cases, the precise meaning of the cancer in Thanos's life will be unique to him. This does not mean that 'anything goes' or that Thanos cannot be mistaken, since close friends and family can still *advise* him on the best course of action, given who Thanos is and what is important to him. But this notion of the 'best' is very different from some objective medical understanding. This 'personal' aspect of risk is to be contrasted with the 'public' aspect of risk and reasonable behaviour that is presupposed by the legal concepts of negligence and recklessness. On the boundary between the personal and the public is the thorny question of whether, in the context of a public healthcare system, to somehow hold smokers responsible for their smoking-related health problems.

With genetic conditions, there is a different kind of risk at stake because the patient might not yet have any symptoms. Does patient autonomy include the right 'not to know', or would this be irresponsible to oneself and to one's dependents? Ruth Stirton begins with questions such as these, and the way that they challenge the general assumption that more information is always a good thing. Part of the problem is the essentially familial nature of genetic illness, so that knowledge of my own condition will sometimes reveal something about my sister's or cousin's condition, thereby generating a new dilemma. In addition, there is the question of whether such information should be relevant to reproductive decisions. These will again be very personal decisions for the people involved, and Stirton is interested in the way such people make sense of the problems and of what might be 'for the best'. She goes on to argue that philosophical engagement with the patient's experience is fundamental to our understanding of genetic illness. She illustrates how phenomenology has been, and could be used to further explore the meaning of genetic illness to the individual patient. This becomes increasingly important as these inherently personal cases are to be contrasted with such public questions of whether health insurance companies (especially in the American context) and employers have a right to use predictive genetic information.

Part IV. The law, the profession and ethics

The first three parts have focused more on the patient, and this last part focuses more on the doctor (and to a certain extent on other healthcare professionals). But instead of asking what the legal, professional and ethical duties of the doctor should be, it asks what doctors *make*, and ought to make, of the duties placed upon them, and how they fulfil such duties in practice. There is also the question of the relationship between the three kinds of duties.

Richard Huxtable looks at the confusions in English law revealed by the case of Charlotte Wyatt, born in 2003 with severe organ problems. On several occasions she was given a very bleak prognosis, and the medical team wanted to implement a Do-Not-Attempt-Resuscitation (DNAR) order. But each time her parents would not agree, so the matter was repeatedly submitted to the courts. While the law is fairly clear in describing the relevant ethical factors, it is less clear in determining the precise content and relative weight of those factors. In Charlotte's case, it was not clear what her 'best interests' were, whether her situation was sufficiently 'intolerable', when the presumption in favour of life has been 'rebutted', or how much weight her parents' wishes should have. The courts vainly hoped that the medical team could resolve the matter by 'discussion' with the parents, without it being clear enough how such a discussion (or rather persuasion) would transpire. Through this all, Charlotte continued to live, and as of 2009 had been out of hospital for two years. Huxtable uses this case and others to ask what can be reasonably expected from the law, both by the public and by doctors; he detects inherent ethical and thus legal indeterminacy and so his cautious suggestion is to make more use of clinical ethics committees.

Cliona McGovern examines the Codes of Ethics that all professions have voluntarily adopted (in particular she looks at medicine and physiotherapy). Such codes have a curious status. They are not law, nor are they part of the legal system; indeed McGovern gives us examples where the courts explicitly returned an issue to the profession for adjudication. Codes of Ethics are not normally considered to be among the body of rules and standards that serve to define the profession, although they approach the implicit standards of professionalism. But because of this ambiguity, there are many professionals who regard them as mere window-dressing. But this status is changing in interesting ways, writes McGovern. In a recent Irish case, two doctors were deemed professionally incompetent for failing to meet expected standards (the so-called 'Bolam test'), but the case examined whether this should have happened at all. The judge found that if the Medical Council had wanted to sanction the doctors, then they should have used the 'moral turpitude' test. At the same time, McGovern describes one area of medical training where the Code of Ethics is flouted with dangerous impunity. Despite the code's explicit requirement to seek the patient's full informed consent, there is enough evidence of anaesthetized patients being used by medical students – at their consultant's behest and pressure – to practice intimate examinations.

Mark Wicclair considers the position of doctors and pharmacists who refuse, for reasons of conscience, to authorize or perform or provide a lawful service, for example, for abortion or emergency contraception. At first glance, such refusals are curious: unlike military conscripts, these professionals all volunteered for training and for work, and they knew well that these services were lawful. And even within the medical profession, there are plenty of jobs (dermatology, pathology) that do not come close to abortion. Doctors and pharmacists are expected to perform other unpleasant tasks and to overcome other kinds of objection, for example those based on nausea or racism. So why the special exemptions granted to conscientious objectors? Why the absence of something like the 'alternative service' that is required from

Chapter 1

The Body: Property, Commodity or Gift?[1]

Alastair V. Campbell

Why the Body Matters

In their evidence into the Inquiry into Alder Hey Children's Hospital, the parents of a girl whose organs had been removed without their knowledge or consent graphically expressed their outrage:

> They were devastated to hear that their daughter's tongue had been retained, and father protested silently outside Alder Hey ... They describe the hospital as having stolen their daughter's body, which was 'white as driven snow'. It was reduced to skin and bone by predators and it must never happen again. (*Royal Liverpool Children's Inquiry* 2001 p. 421)

These words of anger and despair are just one of many examples of how the medical profession failed to appreciate the significance of the bodies of the deceased to their families – and most especially of children – uncovered by this and other investigations and by the work of the Retained Organs Commission, set up by the government in the UK to deal with the aftermath of public inquiries in Liverpool and Bristol. It revealed a gulf of misunderstanding between the medical scientific community and the lay public about why the body matters, whether before or after death. This is well illustrated by evidence given to the Chief Medical Officer's Summit on Organ Retention (2001) by some of the representatives of medical bodies:

> The fact that in the past many families have not been informed in detail about what a post mortem examination entails ... invariably reflected a simple and understandable wish to spare them further anguish and distress at the time of bereavement. (Royal College of Pathologists, ref. 101)

It is perhaps a paradox that in an age when we have more understanding than ever before of the nature of human life and the biology of the human body, we are more distressed than at any time in human history

> about what is perceived as inappropriate disposal of the whole human body or part of it ... This is a philosophical puzzle ... (President, Royal College of Paediatrics and Child Health, ref. 119)

Perhaps this last quotation is the most powerful indication of the narrative dissonance of the medical and lay understandings of the body. The President of the Royal College of Paediatrics and Child Health cannot understand how, with such improved knowledge of the *biology* of the body, relatives can feel distressed when they discover that they have buried a body 'stripped of organs'.

Such a clash of narratives is not restricted to the medical world. The philosopher John Harris shows similar puzzlement and disapproval when considering the controversy over organ retention and the proposals for a more respectful treatment of human remains, describing the reactions of the relatives in harsh terms: '... the complaint of those who object to actions that violate the physical integrity of the corpse is scarcely rational' (Harris 2002 p. 548). Why not rational? Because the body inevitably disintegrates soon after death and 'may end up as a bung in a beer barrel or mortar in a wall' (2002 p. 547).

In a later article, discussing methods of procuring cadaveric organs, Harris has no hesitation in describing the attitudes of those who want to retain bodily integrity after death as 'wicked', because it stands in the way of medical science, which can save the lives of others:

> ... it is surely implausible to think that having one's body remain whole after their death is an objective anyone is entitled to pursue at the cost of other people's lives! It is implausible to the point of wickedness, not least because the objective is irrational and impossible of achievement (Harris 2003 p. 133).

So what has gone wrong here? Is the problem, as Harris and some of the medical experts seem to imply, that the lay public is merely ignorant, selfish and over-emotional? This is both philosophically naïve and insulting – for (as I know from being Vice-Chairman of the Retained Organs Commission), many of the offended parents were highly educated. So far as being over-emotional is concerned, it is hard to see why parents who have suffered the double blow of the unexpected death of a child and deception about the fate of their child's body should not appropriately feel emotion. Nor is it simply the failure to inform parents that is the source of anger and distress. For many parents, those parts which were removed and retained carried a very powerful symbolic force, quite unrecognized by the pathologists excising and retaining the organs. For example, the removal of the child's tongue, referred to in the opening quotation of this chapter, was especially painful for the parents, since their daughter had struggled to learn to speak despite her disabilities. The heart, for many lay people, carries particular resonance, as is evident from this quotation from the evidence to the Bristol Inquiry:

> If they had asked us whether they could retain Lewis's heart for whatever reason we would have said no because we believe the heart is the soul of the person (Janis Wilcox, mother of Lewis, *Bristol Royal Infirmary Inquiry* 2000 paras. 134–140)

As Michaela Willis (herself an affected parent) and I wrote:

> The physical body of the person loved is fully part of the love that parent feels for child or wife for husband. This embodiment of the person does not suddenly disappear in death, though, of course, it soon becomes necessary to let go of the body and live only with the memory and mental images of the person now dead. A mother cuddling her dead child, a husband kissing the cold brow of his wife's dead body, are not acts which *deny* the death of the person. They are part of the story of human lives shared and of the pain, which comes from parting (Campbell and Willis 2006 p. 126).

Behind this failure to appreciate the significance of emotion tied to close personal relationships there lies a whole philosophical tradition. It is the same tradition (as we shall see later), which perceives no difficulty in treating the human body and its parts as commodities to be traded, as part of a person's material possessions. In this tradition the conscious, reasoning mind is the distinctively human part of the person: the body, as the mere container of the mind, has no significance in itself, and the emotions, which can be seen as little more than instinctive bodily reactions, may act as serious impediments to the clear functioning of the mind. Thus, in this view, human value resides wholly in our reasoning capacity; rationality becomes the sole arbiter of ethics.

The power of this approach in creating modern scientific medicine cannot be underestimated. It desacralized the human body, allowing it to be studied as one would any complex mechanism, without fear of this being an affront to human dignity and without need of divine sanction. Anatomical dissection was at the forefront of this new understanding of how the healthy body works and of the pathological factors, which lead to disease and dysfunction. As the science of anatomy slowly freed itself from opposition by the church and from its disreputable association with body snatching and murder (see Richardson 1987), the foundations were laid for an empirically based medical practice, following scientific principles of investigation and testing out therapies by experimental methods, rather than by clinical anecdote and prejudice.

In his remarkable book, *The Birth of the Clinic*, Michel Foucault describes the emergence of clinical medicine as the advent of a new kind of medical 'gaze' (*regard*), which 'sees' the disease beneath the visible surface of the human body. The scientific doctor has a special knowledge gained from the reading of clinical signs, whose meaning has been discovered by the science of pathology. Thus death has illuminated life. Foucault quotes the nineteenth-century pathologist, Bichat: 'Open up a few corpses: you will dissipate at once the darkness that observation alone could not dissipate'. Foucault comments: '... the whole dark underside of disease came to light, at the same time illuminating and eliminating itself like night' (1975 p. 195).

It is now easy to see how the failure to recognize the affront of the removal of organs could be regarded as compassionate medical practice, sparing the relatives (and the doctors – or perhaps *especially* the doctors!) the distraction of strong emotion. Leder has summarized this attitude well, as 'medicine's preference for the corpse':

> Modern medicine, profoundly Cartesian in spirit, has continued to use the corpse as a methodological tool and a regulatory ideal. Medical education begins with the cadaver, just as the clinical case ends with the patho-anatomical dissection (1990 p.146).

In this environment, when the machine-like qualities of the body can best be seen (since there are no distractions from a living person), it is a short step to disregarding the personal significance of the body, to both the person to whom it belongs and to those who treasure that body as an essential feature of the person they love. We have reached the logical outcome of Descartes' insistence that *res cogitans* and *res extensa* are two utterly distinct aspects of reality – the mind is the 'ghost in the machine' (Ryle 1949).

So, a first prerequisite of seeing the true value of the body (whether to patients or to doctors) is to find a more adequate philosophical theory of embodiment. Here the writings of the neurophysiologist, Antonio Damasio, may offer some help. Damasio mapped philosophical discussions of personal identity onto the latest findings about the relationships between consciousness and the pre-conscious functioning of the nervous system. He argues strongly that attempts to separate the mind from the body are scientifically incoherent. His arguments are complex and quite technical in parts, but he presents a fairly accessible account of the mind–body interaction in his popular work, *The Feeling of What Happens*. Of great relevance to the problems raised by the Cartesian disjunction between mind and body is Damasio's account of the emotions, in their distinctively human form, as a constant interplay between the way we think and the way we feel. In a powerful passage, which is worth quoting at length, he describes this interaction:

> At first glance there is nothing distinctively human about emotions, since it is clear that so many nonhuman creatures have emotions in abundance; and yet there is something quite distinctive about the way in which emotions have become connected to the complex ideas, values, principles and judgments that only humans can have, and in that connection lies our legitimate sense that human emotion is special. Human emotion is not just about sexual pleasures or the fear of snakes. It is also about the horror of witnessing suffering and about the satisfaction of seeing justice served; about delight at the sensuous smile of Jean Moreau or the thick beauty of words and ideas in Shakespeare's verse; about the world weary voice of Dietrich Fischer-Dieskau singing Bach's *Ich habe genug*. . . (1999 p. 22).

Damasio's powerful description makes the point that the very core activities of self-consciousness and valuing, so central to rationalist accounts of the self, can be described adequately only if we see the inseparability of bodily based emotion from thought and judgment in ourselves and others. Of course, this is not to ignore the risk that emotions can prejudice our judgment, nor is it to subscribe to some kind of Humean notion that the reason is the 'slave of the passions' (Hume 1911 p. 127). The point is rather that a highly intellectualist account of what we mean by 'valuing' in a moral sense simply does not accord with the way we are, as embodied selves, in which bodily experience and emotional response play a vital part.

To return to the retained organs controversy, we cannot separate this bodily based emotionally rich self from the centrality of relationships with others in our moral lives. The lone rational decider, emerging from a stark rationalistic individualism rooted in Cartesian Dualism, is a parody of the moral agent in real life. It is in our *interdependency* that we find our moral compass and our moral worth, not in some isolated mental space in which 'right' choices are made. This is because, as humans, both bodily and emotional interdependency are the core experiences of our lives, from birth to death. In an earlier publication I described this core human experience as follows:

> To be a creature is to be born of others, to know ourselves through them, to depend on them and create dependency, to know the pain of losing them and finally to be the instance of that pain to others (Campbell 1984 p. 96).

These are essentially bodily experiences, most obviously in infancy, but also as adult relationships are formed, and more obviously again as old age and approaching death make the bodily and emotional ministrations of others ever more important. (For philosophers this is perhaps nowhere more vividly seen than in the life of Iris Murdoch, as this powerfully rational person became ever more dependent on the loving care of her partner.)

It is for these reasons that accusations of 'irrationality' and 'wickedness' against the relatives involved in the retained organs controversy are so simplistic and philosophically shallow. Of course many of the parents, if asked, would have wanted to ensure that some good would come out of their loss. This is clear from evidence, like the following, to the Bristol Inquiry:

> While I was in the waiting room someone asked if they could do a post mortem and I agreed. I thought that, as there was nothing that could be done for Scott, I might as well try and help others. I was not asked about donation or about organ retention. (Evidence from Josephine Player, *Bristol Royal Infirmary Inquiry* 2000 paras. 134–140)

Yet there were other parents for whom such a resolution of their grief would probably not have been possible, since the thought of the dismemberment of their children's bodies, even for therapeutic purposes, was more than they could bear. Respect for all of the relatives involved would have given them the *choice* to receive the return of a whole body or to donate parts of it willingly in the hope of helping others. The concealment of the post mortem practices current at the time left no space for such a moral choice. Instead, a misplaced medical paternalism led to all the bodies being treated as a mere objects for scientific study, as material of use and significance only because of its potential medical utility. This clash of approaches to the ethics of organ retention leads us to broader questions about uses of the body and its parts, whether before or after death. If we have this essential interdependency, related to our embodiment as persons, then how are we to view the body itself? Is it correct to see the body as akin to a material possession? And what moral consequences flow from the different ways in which we may value the body?

My Body, My Property?

We begin with the question of ownership of the body. In what sense, if any, is it correct to describe people's bodies as their property, akin to other material goods, which they may clearly own, such as their houses, goods and chattels, stocks and shares, etc.? It turns out that the concept of property is a complex one, made up of a set of legal (or, possibly, ethical) conditions, all or most of which need to be satisfied in order for us to describe something as genuinely my property. A comprehensive list has been offered by Honoré (1961), comprising eleven types of legal relationship, which might be included in the description of an object as 'my property'. Honoré sees a 'family resemblance' between these eleven features, but does not suggest that all must apply in order for the term to be meaningfully used. Rather, the list provides us with a range of relationships between an object and its owner, which can be applied flexibly to a range of situations of ownership. The following is a brief summary of Honoré's list:

1. *The right to possess* – that is, to have exclusive physical control of the thing
2. *The right to use*
3. *The right to manage*
4. *The right to income*
5. *The right to capital* – that is, the right to alienate the possession by means of sale, mortgage or gift and the right to destroy it
6. *The right to security* – the right to indefinite possession
7. *Transmissibility* – the object can be passed on to the holder's successors or heirs, and so on indefinitely
8. *Absence of term* – no time limit on the ownership
9. *Duty to prevent harm* – either by owner's use of it, or by use of it by others

10. *Liability to execution* – the object possessed can legitimately be removed to settle a debt or deal with insolvency
11. *Residuarity* – the object, if no longer owned by possessor (for example, if abandoned by him) may be owned by others.

This list may seem unduly complicated, and other simpler ones have been suggested. For example, the philosopher, Sidgwick (1891), suggested just three features that constitute ownership – the right to exclusive use, the right to destroy, and the right to alienate. However, the more complex descriptions of Honoré are illuminating for the discussion of whether the body or any of its parts may be appropriately regarded – *in some senses at least* – as property. Which parts of Honoré's bundle seem appropriately attached to the body and its parts?

Let us consider first those parts of the list that *do* seem to apply appropriately to the relationship between me and my body. These are items 1, 2 and 3 relating to exclusive possession and use, and items 6, 8 and 9 relating to unlimited possession and my duty to prevent harm from use. It would be very odd to suppose that such rights and obligations, which apply material property such as my home or my car, do not equally apply to my body and its parts.

But what of those rights which apply to transfer or removal of my property – transmissibility, liability to execution and residuarity? It is clear that while I am alive my body as a whole cannot be treated as capable of being removed from me (alienable) – I cannot transfer it to my heirs; I cannot abandon it, leaving it for others to gain possession; nor can it be removed from me in settlement of a debt. However, I can arrange for the removal and transfer parts of my body, for example, one of my kidneys or some of my blood, and these parts then become, in the senses noted above, property of the recipient. (I cannot demand the return of the donated kidney, claiming it as still my property, once it is transplanted into another person.) After my death transfer of the body or its parts becomes even more viable. The law allows my next of kin to have 'lawful possession' of the body, though only for the purposes of proper disposal of it.

Given adequate consents, parts of my dead body may be removed and transferred to the bodies of others – obvious examples being transplantable corneas and kidneys. Thus these items in Honoré's list do seem to apply, at least to some extent, to my body, in whole or in part.

However, the remaining items on the list, relating to income and capital, are the most contentious, since they equate the body and its parts with commodities, and it is here that the main disagreement about the status of the body as property arises. Given that Honoré allows a flexible view of the concept of property, we may be able to say that, in some senses, our bodies and their constituent parts *are* our property. But in reaching this conclusion, we do not in fact solve the moral problem at the heart of the debate about a commercial trade in body parts. To deal with this, we have to look more deeply at the concept of ownership as it relates to our embodied selves.

Limitations to the property paradigm

There are several reasons for seeing the language of property or ownership, when extended to include trading in body parts, as misleading and unhelpful morally. Firstly, as we saw earlier, we do not 'possess' our whole living body as we might possess some other material thing, for example, a set of clothes. We can remove our clothes, sell them, use them as barter for different items, give them to a charity shop, or simply throw them away. None of this is possible in relation to our bodies, at least when we are alive. (We can alienate parts of our body, but not our body as a whole.) Indeed, as we argued earlier there is no 'we' without our bodies. So, to alienate our bodies, we would have to alienate ourselves, for example, through suicide or voluntary slavery. And there is a second problem in the concept of the body as our exclusive property. As Herring and Chau (2007 p. 45) point out, 'Our bodies are not in any straightforward sense "ours". They are interdependent, interconnected and intermingling with other bodies'. This is true from conception onwards. We are in constant dependency upon, and interaction with, the living environment, and from this relationship we gain life itself. This is at its most obvious in the fetal–maternal relationship during pregnancy, but it continues throughout our lives, right up to the moment of our death.

Every moment of our lives is lived in (mostly unconscious) total dependency on our environment. We are separate beings only in a very restricted sense. Thus, it may be misleading to equate our relationship with our bodies to the relationship we have with our material possessions. Like all living beings, there is no watertight 'oursness' (as Herring and Chau put it) kept within the boundaries of our bodies – life constantly flows back and forward between ourselves, other selves and the environment in which we maintain our existence. Maintaining our bodily integrity within this state of dynamic interactiveness demands procedures quite different from those which help to defend us from trespass into our home or theft of our material possessions.

But, even if the body *as a whole* should not be seen as a tradable commodity, can we perhaps retain the concept to describe people's rights to sell *parts* of their body? For example, Lori Andrews, in an article (misleadingly) entitled 'My body, my property' (1986 p. 37), seems to believe that we can safely distinguish between the whole and the parts:

> It is time to start acknowledging that people's body parts are their personal property. This is distinguishable from the past characterizations of people as property, which were immoral because they failed to take into account the non-bodily aspects of the individual ... and they created rights of ownership by others ... Allowing people to transfer and sell their own body parts, while protecting them from coercion, does not present these dangers.

In the context of the worldwide shortage of solid organs for transplantation, many bioethics writers (Radcliffe-Richards *et al.* 1998; Erin and Harris 2003; Wilkinson 2003) seem to agree with this claim and argue that there is no real ethical problem in our becoming sellers of kidneys (and presumably of other 'disposable' bodily parts), provided it is in a 'regulated market'.

The body bazaar

There is, however, a strangely irresponsible naïveté in the notion that there can be an ethical market in human body parts. The body and its parts have become big business. With the rapid expansion of transplantation of organs and tissues, the development of cell technology and immunosuppressant drugs and the hope of ever new therapeutic marvels from targeted pharmaceuticals, all human material has become of increasing interest to the health care industry. We have seen the emergence of what Andrews and Nelkin (2001) have called the 'body bazaar', in which all forms of human tissue gain commercial significance. At its extreme this bazaar is also bizarre, not to say macabre, reminiscent of the historical trade in dead bodies so well described by Ruth Richardson in *Death, Dissection and the Destitute* (1987). For example, just before Christmas 2005 it was discovered that the leg bones of the journalist, Alistair Cooke, had been removed from his corpse and sold for more than $7,000 to a company making dental implants (Waltz 2006). Clearly the Cooke case is an extreme example, involving absence of consent, deception and (possibly) theft. But what if there had been full consent by Cooke prior to his death and no deception? Would it be ethically acceptable for people to include as part of their legacy authorized sale of their bodily 'assets'? It could be their most valuable asset and could perhaps relieve the concerned dependents from destitution! And, if this would be acceptable after death, why not equally during life? Can we ethically view our body and its parts as a tradable resource, to be removed and sold for financial gain, if we so choose?

There are both consequentialist and in-principle objections to such a proposal. The consequentialist ones concern the inevitability of exploitation. In any such market the poor will always be the principal, or possibly the sole, sellers, while in most societies it is the rich who will gain the benefits without taking the risks. Moreover, in this market, the poor, far from being rescued from their desperate state, as Radcliffe-Richards *et al.* (1998) assert, end up being worse off.[2]

The in-principle objections flow from my earlier discussion of the inseparability of the body from the integrity of the person. It is no argument to say that just because there is an illegal market in organs, our only recourse to the evident need for such organs to save lives is to attempt to introduce a regulated market. Let us take an obvious example: it is a correct description to say that there has been (and probably still is) a market in slaves, just as there is ample evidence of a continuing market in child sex workers. However, the fact that vulnerable adults and children are *in fact* treated as commodities, does not mean that it is *morally justifiable* to treat them in this way.

Of course, it might be argued that in any instance of the use of persons as mere means, we need to assess the relative harms and benefits. So, while the harm of treating children as sex objects cannot be outweighed by any benefits to the overall happiness of society – though some might contest this – there will be other cases where the benefits are clear. Thus organ trading can save lives and also might bring financial benefit to the donor. Here, however, we have a direct clash of moral theory. A consequentialist might offer the example of a desperate father selling himself into slavery in order to raise enough money to feed his family, at least for a few months. If the balance of benefit over harm is positive, why would this be wrong? But the in-principle objection regards this as wholly unacceptable. No beneficial consequences can justify treating persons as the possessions of others, as tradable items, whose value can be determined according to the going price in the market. So while principlists may understand such a desperate move, they cannot ever view it as morally right. Underlying this view of the moral wrongness of such commodification of persons is the dictum of Immanuel

Kant that we should always treat moral agents, including ourselves, as ends in themselves, never as mere means.

But, assuming we grant this central moral principle about the moral wrongness of commodifying *persons*, does this prohibition extend to treating the (alienable) *parts of the bodies* of persons as commodities? Here we are in the realm of what Margaret Radin calls 'contested commodities' (Radin 1996). She argues that there are currently powerful political and social forces leading us toward universal commodification of all aspects of persons, including their bodies. This derives from the pervasive influence of a free market philosophy, which in turn is based on 'negative freedom' (Berlin 1958) – the freedom to trade without interference from others or from the state. Radin believes that this assertion of negative freedom is self-defeating, for, how can a person be regarded as free, if at the same time she is regarded as no more than 'a manipulable object of monetizable value (from the point of view of others)' (1996 p. 56)? In opposition to this all-pervasive market ideology, Radin argues for a positive, not a negative, view of freedom – one which emphasizes the need for an enabling community in which the richness of total human flourishing is enhanced by non-market social structures. So, in opposition to the view that persons are merely traders in a 'free' market, Radin describes personhood in these terms:

> ... a better view of personhood should understand many kinds of particulars – one's politics, work, religion, family, love, sexuality, friendships, altruism, experiences, wisdom, moral character, and personal attributes – as integral to the self. To understand any of these as monetizable or completely detachable from the person ... is to do violence to our deepest understanding of what it is to be human (1996 p. 56).

Following Radin, we can see that opposition to encouraging a trade in human body parts relates to the quality of our community life. It takes us back to the same central ethical issue arising from the retained organs controversy, in which the final affront was the depersonalization of the dead children's bodies and the lost opportunity for the bereaved parents to be treated as willing and committed partners in the quest to prevent such tragedies in the future. The moral texture of voluntary donation (of parts of myself or of my deceased relatives) is utterly different from the competitive values of 'the body bazaar'. We are once again at a clash of moral perspectives in this assessment of the values at stake. Returning to John Harris's accusation of 'wickedness' described earlier in this chapter, some might see this opposition to commodification as a morally irresponsible approach, since (allegedly, at least) allowing trade in organs could save many lives. But the question remains, what is the cost to our communal lives will such an acceptance of the ubiquity of the market entail?

Another Country – Giving to Unnamed Strangers

My argument to this point inevitably leads to a classic work on the philosophy of altruistic donation, *The Gift Relationship* by Richard Titmuss, first published in 1970. Titmuss takes us to another country from the one described by Radin (and which we seem increasingly to inhabit), where *everything* has its price. For Titmuss a society's worth depended on how it treated the needs of 'unnamed strangers', and this high social value was classically enshrined in the voluntary donation of blood. Titmuss's claims have been the subject of prolonged and intense debate in the forty years since the book was published, and in the scope of this chapter it is possible only to give a sense of the main issues. What is important to note, however, is that the argument espoused by Titmuss is not restricted to blood donation, but can be applied equally to all forms of possible commodification of the body and its parts.

The essence of his approach is captured in the subtitle of the book: *From human blood to social policy*. Titmuss is concerned with fundamental questions about the creation of an ideal human community in which the lives of all citizens are both protected and enriched. At the time when he was doing the research for the book he was concerned about the encroachment of a market philosophy into all aspects of social policy, including the provision of health care (an even more topical concern today!). For him, a society which fails to foster altruism and a real sense of communal responsibility and which fails to counter the natural human propensity to selfishness is doomed to moral chaos and the collapse of humane social structures. Acquisitiveness and greed will easily gain social dominance unless we create the kind of social arrangements that motivate us to care for others. The voluntary donation of blood is simply a powerful example of how altruism can be encouraged and the dangers of the market philosophy effectively countered.

David Archard, in a careful philosophical analysis of Titmuss's argument, calls it the 'transformative claim' (Archard 2002 p. 89). In its negative aspect, it sees the market as having a contaminating effect on altruism – 'eroding community and repressing altruism', to use Titmuss's words. The contaminating effect of the market could work in two ways: first, the *meaning* of my gift would be changed, since there is now a market price for blood (or other tissues). Rather than seeing it as the gift of life to a needy stranger, I now would see myself simply as making a financial contribution to the health service, waiving the financial claim I could have made for providing the blood. This would still be a gift, of course, but its meaning, according to this argument, is impoverished. Since blood is the stuff of life itself, to equate it to a financial sum is to denude it of its symbolic value. Secondly, now that blood has been given a financial value, my *motivation* to give would be removed, for why should I need to donate when hospitals can obtain commercially the blood required to care for patients? Further, why donate something when I can sell it instead?

Some writers have questioned the force of this negative claim. For example, Mack (1989) points to examples where a market price and a genuine gift easily co-exist. I may give my wife a sweater worth (say) $50 and also donate to my injured friend a pint of blood, whose market price might also be $50, but in both cases the gift is uncontaminated by the fact it has a market value. This is because it is not the monetary value that is crucial here, but my expression of love or concern for the recipient.

However, this argument, as Archard points out, works only when *closely personal* relationships are involved. Of course, my wife and my friend perceive the value of the gift, not in monetary terms, but in terms of my careful choice of it, which demonstrates my appreciation of them as persons; and neither they, nor I, would see the value of the gift as diminished, simply because it has a monetary equivalent. But these modifying features do not apply outside the sphere of such special, personal relationships. The whole point of Titmuss's argument is that my altruistic act expresses my sense of obligation to *strangers* (and to the community as a whole), and this sense of social responsibility and commitment to the welfare of others does not come naturally – it needs fostering (so Titmuss believes) by being clearly separated from commercial equivalents.

We return once more to the centrality of relationships in any consideration of the moral significance of the body and its parts. Some of these may be close personal ones, as when I donate an organ to a friend or relative in dire need: others, may be quite distant, and in essence anonymous, as when I sign a form authorizing the removal of my organs after death for use by needy others, or when I donate my blood to a bank to be universally available, according to need alone. This is the 'other country', in which I am not in any sense a trader and in which I cannot ever calculate the relative balance of loss and gain, to ensure that I have done a good deal.[3]

Conclusions

I began this chapter with the powerful emotions raised by the retained organs controversy and by the uncomprehending medical and philosophical reaction to these wholly justified emotions. I have ended it with the debate about whether much needed bodily tissues, such as blood and organs, should be voluntarily donated or traded in some kind of regulated market. There is a common theme throughout. This is the centrality of relationships in a moral evaluation of the significance of the human body. I believe this theme to be an absolutely crucial one in the further development of medical ethics, as technological breakthroughs offer more and more options for using and modifying the human body. There is increasingly powerful political pressure on the medical profession to set up collaborations with the biotechnological industry and to become involved in the kind of research that will ensure both escalating profits and patentable inventions. In all *furor economicus* the core values of medicine are at serious hazard. No longer does medicine become a moral enterprise, which puts the suffering person at its centre and which campaigns for a society in which all members are treated with equal respect and with a proportionate concern for their needs. In its place we find the patient as a consumer in the health care market and the body as a commodity, giving competitive advantage or disadvantage to the individual. A medical *ethics* worthy of its name must surely be devoted to reversing this descent into moral anarchy.

Chapter 2

Ricœur's Medical Ethics: The Encounter Between the Physician and the Patient

Gaëlle Fiasse

Dedicated to Paul Bouvier

In this chapter, I will use the contemporary ethics of Paul Ricœur and his specific articles on medicine in order to focus on the patient–doctor relationship. More specifically, I will explain the structure of what Ricœur calls his 'little ethics' and I will apply it to the specific case of medicine. Ricœur's ethics not only refers to norms and prohibitions (the deontological aspect of morality), but it also comprises a meta-ethic, a reflection on norms that refers to, in Ricœur's own words, 'the ethical aim of the good life'.[1] In order to come back to the origin of the norms, Ricœur constantly uses Aristotelian ethics, and he revisits some notions such as desire (*orexis*), ultimate goal (*telos*), happiness (*eudaimonia*), and prudential judgement (*phronèsis*). While reading such concepts, it should be kept in mind that they have a particular Greek resonance which has given rise to a long history of commentary in Continental philosophy.[2]

At the end of this chapter, I will show how two other Ricœurian concepts can help us to better highlight the relationship between patients and medical workers. The first is the recognition of oneself as another fragile person in Ricœur's anthropology of the capable and suffering human being. The second is the mode of translation where learning to speak the 'language' of the other can be interpreted as a proper mode of being with others.

Before getting into great detail, it is worth noting that Ricœur's work on ethics and medicine has not been referenced much by philosophers who have published anthologies on biomedical ethics in North America.[3] His specific work on *ethics and medicine* seems absent for the most part in biomedical ethics, even within the medical community. Paradoxically, there is a gap between the absence of his proper ethics applied to medicine and an increasing interest in his other publications on *literature and hermeneutics* within the medical community, especially in nursing ethics and narrative medicine. Narrative medicine, contrary to principlism and casuistry, focuses on narrative competence to recognize and interpret the stories of patients[4]. It counters the reduction of medicine to a techno-science or a mere interpretation of scientific data, and it promotes the use of literature in the training of medical students to help them to reflect on suffering, death, disease, and healing. A component of narrative medicine is storytelling which is used as a conceptual tool to help patients to recount the story of their lives, such as teenagers who constrain their identities to being anorexic or patients in search of meaning and identity when they have difficulties in coping with the loss of health. In this sense, Ricœur's notion of 'narrative identity', which counters a rigid identity and integrates changes and the role of others in one's own life story, is used more and more in Europe and North America as a tool to help drug addicts, patients with a psychosis, people suffering from cancer, etc.[5] I will, however, not develop the theme of narrative identity *per se*, but rather focus on another aspect of Ricœur's work which deserves closer attention: the pact of care between a doctor and a patient.

Ricœur's 'Little Ethics' and the Case of Medicine

Ethics as preceding the moral norms

Ricœur stresses that the first question in moral philosophy is not 'What ought I to do?' but 'How would I like to lead my life?' What does this mean concretely for an agent? It means that before turning to the imperatives that belong to common morality such as 'Do not kill', 'Do not lie', or to other maxims (which must be put to the test of universalization), an agent should act not only out of respect for duty, but because he discovers that what motivates his moral actions are also his highest 'expectations'. Applied to medicine, this notion of 'expectation' is of crucial importance, since Ricœur connects 'our ordinary expectations, however controversial they may be', with 'the notion of health as a form of well-being and happiness' (Ricœur 2007f pp. 199–200). Norms are rooted in life and in human desire (*orexis*).

Thus for Ricœur, the three major points that delineate an 'ethics' which precedes a 'morality' are 'the aim of a good life (i), with and for another (ii), in just institutions (iii)'. These three aspects correspond respectively to the self (i), the other (ii) and the 'third' (iii) understood as those 'left outside of the face-to-face encounter of an I and a you' (Ricœur 2002 p. 195). First, every human being aims at a fulfilling life. Second, what gives an orientation to one's actions is to do something not only with another person but also for another person. This dimension 'with and for another' refers to the relationships of proximity, that is, those of solicitude. Solicitude relates to mutuality, that is, to a kind of friendship where both friends discover each other as unique and irreplaceable. It is 'the structure common to all these dispositions favourable towards others that underlie the nearby relations of intersubjectivity' (Ricœur 2007b p. 53). Third, given that we do not live an isolated life, all relationships of proximity are also lived in a broader context, that is, in interaction with other people who are not individuals we meet in 'face-to-face' relationships. Just institutions, which can include each person, therefore constitute this third aspect. The most evident feature of our commitment to just institutions is our participation in political institutions.

Ethics is defined by an aim in the sense that we have a goal towards which we direct our actions, even though it is only under the 'optative' mode of *wishing* to live well, wishing to live with and for another, and finally wishing to live in just institutions. It can be a goal beyond our scope, but still a guiding ideal.

Let us illustrate this three-pronged ethics of Ricœur's in the case of medicine by starting with the first point: *aiming at a good life.* According to Ricœur, 'medical ethics is inscribed within the general ethics of living well and of living together' (Ricœur 2000a p. 25). Medical practitioners share with their patients the same wish, which is physical and mental health. They are first and foremost human beings dealing with other human beings who are suffering. The fact that ethics precedes morality means that the precepts physicians follow have their roots in human desire (*orexis*). To put it more simply, behind all rules and interdictions there lies a value to be discovered. Furthermore, it means that being a good doctor, for instance, also concerns fulfilling a *practice.* The self evaluates himself or herself according to rules which precede him or her. Every profession is shaped by the standards of excellence attached to the profession. In this sense, the Hippocratic oath continues to bind doctors even today (*ibid.* p. 24).

The second aspect of Ricœur's ethics concerns the good life *with and for another.* Both the patient and the physician are partners of a common struggle against illness (Ricœur 2007g p. 215). Medical practitioners have to care for a *patient* and, in this sense, they are not only curing a disease, or an *interesting case,* but a unique human being. The specific nature of medicine is to be a practice 'based on a social relation for which suffering is the basic motivation' (Ricœur 2007f p. 199). For Ricœur, it is precisely this dimension of solicitude that best illustrates the relationship between a patient and a doctor. Therapeutic practice differs from biological and medical sciences in the laboratory, in that curiosity is not the primary motive, but solicitude or compassion (Ricœur 2007g p. 215). Ricœur speaks about a *pacte de soins* (a 'pact of care', 'treatment pact', 'caregiving agreement'). Rather than being primarily a 'contract' in the deontological sense, the *pact of care* is based on trust and confidentiality as a principal component of medical ethics. Ricœur insists on the fact that the pact of confidentiality has the 'the features of an affinity linking two people in an elective manner' (Ricœur 2007f p. 204). For this reason, confidentiality can be assigned to a feature shared with the virtue of friendship. The pact of care that binds a patient and a physician can *ethically* be seen as a relationship marked by an asymmetry. The patient lives in a condition of fragility and suffering according to which he puts himself into the hands of a doctor who has the power of action. The doctor is the one 'who knows what to do and offers treatment' (Ricœur 2001 p. 115). Ricœur analyzes in detail the pact of care between patient and physician, as well as the different steps of which it is composed which tend to equalize the dissymmetry. The patient starts by describing his symptoms. His complaint includes *a narrative component* which seeks to gather the entangled details. As I said above, Ricœur's notion of narrative identity is one of the most well-known aspects of his anthropology and has been applied in particular to different fields of medicine which emphasize attention to the patient's story and context.[6] After describing his symptoms, the patient formulates a request for a cure, that is, for health. Ricœur stresses the trust on the basis of which the pact of care is formed, even though it can also conceal any mistrust on the part of the patient towards the physician because of the asymmetrical relationship of power and, paradoxically, any excessive trust in the physician's power to heal, marked by the patient's enduring dream of immortality. A 'just distance' (Ricœur 2007g p. 220) is to be found in the relationship between the patient and the doctor, which is not indifference, nor condescension or disregard, but neither it is an emotional fusion where the two identities could be lost. Ricœur mentions the steps from the side of the physician who accepts the patient, formulates a diagnosis, and prescribes a treatment. These steps help to show the concrete pact of care, which is bound by mutual commitments[7] and the 'prescription' which is the recording of this alliance. The patient promises to conduct himself as an agent of the proposed treatment. The doctor commits himself to follow the patient.

As for the third aspect, *living well in just institutions*, the institution at stake is of course the medical profession. In spite of the singular experience between each doctor and each patient, every pact is nonetheless subject to 'the regulations that make up the professional code of ethics governing every medical art' (Ricœur 2001 p. 115). Anyone working in the medical field can meet each patient personally, but each relationship arises in a particular context shaped by the precepts and norms of the medical profession in a particular country.

Morality, asymmetry and the Golden Rule

According to Ricœur, ethics is not sufficient to determine a good moral choice. The reason for this is that there is always the possibility of violence, insofar as our desires can be biased. That is why Ricœur adds morality to ethics, inspired by the Kantian tradition. Imperatives are necessary for countering violence and evil. Interdictions and norms foster our moral duties. Although formalization is often a gain, it can also be a weakness if in the process we lose sight of genuine respect for the individuality of the other person. With Kant, we are placed at a high level of formalization which extends to anyone and requires them to be considered as an end and never as a means. But Ricœur's grounding of morality in solicitude (the ethical component) helps to take into consideration the patient as such, as a person deserving genuine respect. The categorical imperative (the moral component) helps to extend the spirit of solicitude to any patient and to take into account the plurality of persons.

In the medical field, suffering and the request for treatment give rise to the medical act. Accordingly, Ricœur emphasizes that the fundamental norm is the one that obliges:

> the members of the medical profession in general to offer aid not only to their patients but to any sick or wounded person they may come upon in a life-threatening situation. At this level of generality, the duties applying to the medical profession tend to become confused with the categorical imperative to help any person in danger (Ricœur 2007f p. 204. See also Ricœur 2001 p. 116).

Solicitude towards another thus takes the form of a concrete norm. Ricœur also states the norm as follows: 'Every person has the right to be cared for, regardless of social condition, race, ethnicity, religion, customs, or beliefs'.[8] Following the reflections made by Hans Jonas (1979/1992) on technology, Ricœur stresses that every power increases situations of fragility.[9] Every time there is an asymmetry in power, there is also the threat of not respecting others (even though it is done in order to respect the rules).

According to Ricœur, every action is 'a power-over' someone else. Simply, by acting, the agent creates an asymmetry. The Golden Rule which stipulates to treat the other as we would like to be treated can thus help us to see, as if in a mirror, our power-to-act reversed through the possibility of suffering. By putting oneself in the place of the other, the agent can imagine himself as the victim of his own action and can be led to prevent the manifold possibilities of violence. By imagining that the other must be deemed as ourselves, we avoid the gap of considering ourselves as ruling over subordinated people. We overcome the selfish tendency which could lead us to consider only our own interests and nothing else, thus we treat the other with respect. In this sense, the Golden Rule plays an intermediary role between ethics and morality. The Golden Rule is a means of protecting the irreplaceable aspect of the other person discovered in solicitude, and of turning towards a formalization and an imperative.

Practical wisdom or prudential judgement (*Phronèsis*)

For Ricœur, morality cannot supersede ethics, since the application of rules requires a special attention to the other person. For this reason, prudential judgements constitute the third aspect of his developments on ethics. 'Prudential judgement' (*phronèsis*) illustrates the contrast between general rules and 'decisions taken in singular situations'. The term *prudential* does not mean cautious as it does in everyday language. It means rather the *orthos logos*, the right reasoning or practical wisdom applied to the singular case, especially in regard to difficult and tragic decisions, conflicts, and suffering. Ricœur's ethics rests on a tripod: the ethical aim, the moral norms, and 'prudential judgement' or 'practical wisdom' (*phronèsis*).

In the domain of medicine, prudential judgement refers to the kind of judgement doctors make with respect to norms and according to each singular situation of their patients who are suffering. Medical decisions refer not only to moral rules such as the deontological codes in medicine, but also to scientific knowledge and professional expertise. Ricœur even compares the medical field to the magistracy in order to show their similarity, which is that they both 'proceed from a general rule to making a decision regarding concrete situations'(Ricœur 2001 p. 117).

Ultimately, moral *judgements-in-situation* may also involve a phase of taking advice from the most competent and the wisest people, according to the

Greek meaning. In the medical field, the committees of bio-ethics can be a resource for counsel (see Ricœur 1992 p. 273) when ethical challenges are at stake, especially in regards to care for the dying. Ricœur has in mind not only the Clinical Ethics Committees. He also speaks about an 'advisory body' (Ricœur 2007g p. 220) where the medical hierarchy would be flattened from the head physician to the nurses in order to judge better certain situations such as those of patients near the end of life.

Precepts and Norms in Medicine

As we have seen with the anteriority of ethics over morality, Ricœur does not immediately focus on norms that are incumbent upon the members of the medical profession. Rather, he pinpoints the ethical demands that give rise to the norms. For this reason, he also opposes 'precepts' to 'norms'. 'Precepts' belong to *ethics* and to what one discovers in an interpersonal relationship with another person, even if it is close to the meaning of the face of the other who obliges us, as described by Levinas. 'Norms' by contrast, refer to the rules that are written in the *deontological* codes of medicine and to imperatives and prohibitions.[10]

The level of commitment in the pact of care, which requires prudential judgement, is not only a matter of benevolence but a question of practice. 'As any art, practiced case by case, it produces, precisely due to teaching and exercise, what can be called precepts ...' (Ricœur 2000a p. 18). Ricœur mentions *three precepts* attached to the medical profession: singularity, indivisibility, and esteem.

By *singularity*, Ricœur means the irreplaceable character of each patient and the particularity of his situation of care. We might find here part of an answer to the issue of respecting cultural diversity in hospitals, especially in medical systems where the patients cannot choose who examines them. For instance, it can be more difficult for a woman of a particular religion or culture to be examined by a male gynaecologist. This kind of demand especially arises in university hospitals which train students in medicine and are mandated to give them the opportunity to learn. In such cases, the patient is seen by a physician together with one or more advanced students. A request from a woman to not be examined by a male gynaecologist or male student in gynaecology should not be judged as a sexist demand, since it could be seen in light of the nakedness related to intimacy and in light of the natural shame a naked woman can feel in front of a man. In some hospitals, the practice of drawing partial curtains aims at increasing this kind of respect. Regardless of whether we can accommodate cultural diversity, it seems important to keep in mind what Ricœur emphasizes in describing the precept of singularity: 'The diversity of human persons mandates that it is not the species one cares for, but in each case a unique specimen of humankind' (Ricœur 2000a p. 18). However, such a precept should not be isolated from the ethical structure of Ricœur's philosophy (ethical aim, norms, and practical wisdom). Ricœur does not say that physicians should agree with all the individual demands from patients. There is for instance a risk of confusing obligation of care with obligation of results. Imperatives are there to counter biased desires. Respect for the other, grounded in solicitude and strengthened by the categorical imperative, is concerned with respect for patients and respect for doctors. Racist claims from patients should not be accommodated.

If I insist on this point, it is because in a recent article in the *Journal of Medical Ethics* (Killmister 2010 pp. 160–164), a very subjective definition of human dignity, called the 'aspirational dignity' model, has been suggested. Dignity is defined as the 'inherent capacity for upholding one's principles and one's standards'. However, this criterion does not seem very different from the capacity to feel humiliated. Dignity is reduced to experience, according to our own standards and principles. The author of such a view endorses the subjectivity of this criterion to the point of citing as a possible example the dignity of a racist patient who would indeed be 'compromised' if he finds 'the experience of being treated by a black doctor or nurse to be humiliating'. According to this author, such a case of humiliated dignity would not give rise to major difficulties since 'dignity is not the only principle guiding medical practice'. *Pace* such a remark, we might object that a twofold problem occurs when dignity is reduced to such a degree of subjectivity. The first is that it becomes impossible to counter false claims of violated dignity, as the example of the racist patient clearly illustrates. The second problem concerns valid cases where people's dignity is genuinely violated but they are unable to give a voice to it. As Jean-Philippe Pierron expresses it by referring to the incapacity of the power-to-speak exemplified by Ricœur, 'there is a suffering when we cannot say what we feel, the language of complaint (cry, groan) stumbling over the conveying of painful lived experience up to the inexpressible' (Pierron 2010 p. 133; see also Ricœur 1992 pp. 12–13).

This remark on the obstacles to expressing one's capacities leads us to the second precept which is the *indivisibility* of the person. 'It is not multiple organs that are treated but a patient who is, so to speak, whole, one'. This precept is also opposed to the 'split between the biological, the psychological, and the social' (Ricœur 2000a p. 18). Following our example of the person unable to express her suffering, there is a risk of dichotomizing the capacities that are visible from the other dimensions of the person which can become less visible because of a situation of fragility, be it physical or mental. To this second precept of indivisibility, we might object that the surgeon only focuses on the body. Here also the precept of indivisibility can be an ethical guide to answering such an objection, insofar as Ricœur stresses the risk of letting therapeutic medicine be colonized by scientific research when scientific consultations take place during the surgical operation.

The third precept refers to a point very often developed by Ricœur in his ethical articles, namely the concept of *self-esteem*, but here applied to the medical world. This precept focuses on the subject's recognition of his own value. Self-esteem includes a twofold dimension of reflexive and relational, of the self and the other, insofar as self-esteem refers to a relation of oneself to oneself and to 'a claim addressed to others' (Ricœur 2007e p. 196). Even though it can be decreased by situations of dependence, such as in hospitalization or offensive and humiliating behaviour, the reference to a patient's self-esteem is a precept that can guide both patients and anyone from the medical profession insofar as it counters the side effects of the disease as a kind of self-exclusion. Health workers are thus called to compensate for the lack of self-esteem by a 'supplementary or supplementing esteem' (*ibid.* p. 197). At this level, studies on narrative identity become helpful to medical practitioners. Personal identity implies a work of mourning especially applied not only to lost objects such as health, but also to one's desires and projects attached to it. Ricœur stresses that 'it is a double labour of memory and mourning that grafts together the sense of self-esteem' (*ibid.* p. 196). We may link what Ricœur says about the responsibility to compensate for a lack of self-esteem to his insistence on referring to resources of strength that we might find in the handicapped person. Under the form of a question, he raises how to reach, beyond the disease, the resources of the will to live, the will of initiatives, evaluations and decisions. He also mentions the duty attached to any 'supposedly healthy individual' to discern in the handicapped person the resources of 'conviviality, of sympathy, of living with and suffering with' (*ibid.* p. 197).

Besides these three precepts, Ricœur stresses *three norms* that govern the medical consultation. He relates these norms to the deontological aspect of his 'little ethics', the domain of norms and imperatives with the process of universalization. These norms are less closely derived from the irreducible aspect of the other found in solicitude. The three norms are medical secrecy, the patient's right to know the truth, and informed consent. Once again, it is interesting to see them as nonetheless fostering the relationship between a patient and a doctor.

Ricœur has in mind the *French Code of Medical Deontology* for which he wrote the foreword in 1996. What he particularly underlines is the correspondence between the rights and duties of patients and doctors. To the norms defining *medical secrecy* from the doctors' side, there correspond norms governing the *patient's rights to know the truth.* The latter concerns the diagnosis, the proposed treatment, and the likely outcome. Such norms do not erase the use of practical wisdom (*phronèsis*). Consideration must be taken for the patient's capacity to receive and accept truth. One must know also 'how to communicate this truth' (Ricœur 1992 p. 269). Ricœur mentions the particular problem of telling the truth to the dying. Two extremes must be avoided. The first is wielding the clinical truth as a death sentence, that is, telling the truth only with respect for the law without taking into account the capacity of the dying to receive it. The second extreme is knowingly lying 'out of fear, one believes, of weakening the forces in the patient struggling against death' (*ibid.*). For Ricœur, practical wisdom requires a bit of creativity in order to find the just behaviour suited to the other as such, by knowing that there might be exceptions even though it should never consist in 'transforming into a rule the exception to the rule' (*ibid.*). The third norm is *informed consent.* It is situated at the juncture of medical confidentiality and truth, since it also concerns the knowledge and understanding of the risks involved in the treatment.

Problems particularly arise when the art of medicine is replaced by the urge for experimentation, when the human body is treated as a thing, and not as the flesh of a living person. Ricœur highlights *three paradoxes.* First, the human person is not a thing, yet her body is part of physical nature which we can observe. Second, the person is not a form of merchandize, nor part of a business, yet medicine has a cost for society. Third, suffering is private, yet health is public (public health). The privacy of suffering has to do with the 'ultimate refuge of singularity' (Ricœur 2007f p. 199), which is common to the singular aspect of enjoyment. My lived experience of suffering is never the same as yours even if we can suffer from the same loss.

A More Singular and More Universal Attention

In a comparison between the medical sphere and the judicial sphere, Ricœur notices that judgement is also a matter of argumentation and interpretation. The rule needs the work of the imagination, that is, 'inventiveness, originality' (Ricœur 2001 p. 118). Such creativity can serve as the respect for the other as such.

In the same line of thought, Ricœur, in various articles, speaks of a demand for justice to be more universal and more singular, even though such a unification may seem paradoxical. Applied to the other, we can see that attention to the other should be more *universal* in the sense of including every person. This universality touches on the meaning of 'just' institutions. Relationships can be biased, so the challenge is to be just to everybody, whatever our affinities, animosities, and our own hierarchies of values may be.

Besides the universal dimension, Ricœur also suggests a kind of attention that would be more *singular* in the sense of paying attention to the other as such, and not to the other as an anonymous individual with no care for his individuality. In the particular case of medicine, it would mean that health care workers should treat each patient without any exception as a person who has the same value as anybody else, and always as a unique person with special and specific needs and problems. For Ricœur, the concept of solicitude and friendship where both individuals love the other for who the other is, illuminates the ethical aim. Indeed, it is precisely in the solicitude of a face-to-face relationship that I discover the uniqueness of the other and can transpose my concern for the other to what Ricœur calls the 'third person'.

This universal and singular attention is an important contribution to the contemporary debate about human dignity. Human dignity is diminished in contemporary debates when no specific areas of actualization are distinguished, and when actualization means only the technical sense of efficiency, competency, and proof of success, such as in economics. Ricœur, on the contrary, does not limit human dignity to actualization. He insists on the passive side of his definition of the human being as 'acting *and suffering*' in the same way as he qualifies the human being as autonomous *and* fragile. For Ricœur, capacities are more fundamental than fulfilments of them (Ricœur 1992a p. 181); competences more stable than performances (Ricœur 2007c p. 86). He mentions different incapacities related to the powers of the capable person (Ricœur 1992b pp. 12–16), and he stresses the role of the other on the path towards actualization (Ricœur 1992a p. 181). For instance, in order to denounce the violence of some institutions, he shows how historical conditions can stop the development of a person, that is, her actualization.

Oneself as Another Fragile Person and the Phenomenon of Translation

Insistence on the two-sides of 'acting and suffering' leads one to see that the other who is fragile can also be oneself. Ricœur notices that we receive something in particular from the fragile other which is the recognition of our own vulnerability and condition of mortality. In his articles on ethics which are not directly addressed to medicine, Ricœur insists on the fact that helping the other means helping him towards fulfilment and flourishing. He says 'It is towards the future of a being, who must be helped to survive and to grow, that we are directed'.

What seems important to me in such a remark is the way in which we consider fragile people, especially in the situation of care. The problem is not only that of excruciating treatments which aim only at keeping the patient alive, but also the gaze we have on the fragile patient which could be disrespectfully paternalistic if we only stare at fragilities. A particular ethical problem arises with statistical tools that pretend to measure the quality of a person's life by focusing on some strict criteria and neglecting many other dimensions of the person. Sometimes a suffering person can be more actualized in other dimensions of her being than the person treating her. That is why if it is crucial to hear the call from another person who is fragile, there is also a risk of falsely imagining ourselves in the same situation. When we think of all the difficulties we faced in our lives, if we had known of them in advance, we would never have thought that we had the strength to overcome them, even if finally we did cope with them. Something similar can happen when we see people who are suffering and we 'imagine' their situations. One may focus on only one aspect of the other's life which seems to us insurmountable without paying attention to the larger situation.

I will end this article on Ricœur's ethics by applying another aspect of his late writings to the particular case of medicine, namely the phenomenon of translation. In an article on the difference between pain and suffering, Ricœur insists on the incommunicable aspect of suffering. He also relates the capabilities developed in his anthropology to specific incapacities. One consequence of suffering is that it damages our capacity to tell the story of our life through stories that are understandable and acceptable. Suffering can rupture the narrative thread of our lives.

I would thus like to illustrate the relationship medical workers have with their patients in light of Ricœur's late writings on translation. In the same way as a suffering person cannot convey what is incommunicable in her experience, languages can be said to be a priori untranslatable into one another. There is no perfect transition from one language to another. A need arises 'to give up the dream of perfect translation' by admitting 'the unsurpassable difference between what is peculiar to us, what is foreign, so that the test of the foreign remains' (Ricœur 2007d p. 115).

In the same way as we can learn a foreign language, we can try to decipher what the other's needs are by trying to understand what he says even though his experience of suffering can be incommunicable. Translation can thus be seen as an anthropological model for our relationships with the other person, who always remains other than us. Even though translations are never perfect, yet possible, we might say that in a similar way respect for a patient will never be perfect, but always possible, and indeed in the perpetual mode of being improved.

In conclusion, norms and precepts foster the objective duties of the pact of care between patients and doctors, whereas practical judgement and solicitude orient their application by respecting the genuine individuality of the other. The encounter between a physician and a patient can be seen in light of mutual fragilities and as an exercise of translation.

Chapter 3

Bringing the Lived Body to Medical Ethics Education: Learning to See the Suffering Other

Kristin Zeiler

Introduction

Virtue ethical approaches, with their foci on the character of the moral subject, on motivations, emotions and relationships, can enable ethics in medicine and provide fuller ethical examinations and more context-sensitive and creative solutions than can principle-based or consequentialist reasoning alone. Such reasoning can explain the persistent interest with moral virtues in medicine. Virtue ethics is seen as a valuable alternative or complement to other ways of grappling with moral dilemmas in medicine, where a number of principles have been applied to particular cases with some considerations of possible consequences of different actions (see Pellegrino 2001, Bolsin *et al.* 2005, Gardiner 2003, Thomasma 2000, Tong 1998). Though the latter frameworks give valuable ethical insights, they have their limits in terms of how different principles should be valued and weighted against each other.

Virtue ethical approaches are commonly concerned with the subject becoming virtuous. This requires time and continuous practice. It involves habituation. In this regard, the development of virtues shares features with the development of practical skills. In both cases, we learn by doing. Despite the fact that the learning of practical skills is an interest for phenomenologists such as Maurice Merleau-Ponty (2006), surprisingly little dialogue has taken place between virtue ethics and phenomenological traditions.[1] Such a dialogue will arise in this text. A phenomenological analysis can deepen our understanding of how the practical know-how of virtues can feed into the subject's embodied existence and perception. It can throw new light on the debated phenomenon of moral perception. And it can matter for medical ethics education.

A few previous studies have elaborated a phenomenology of virtue that examines what it is like to be a virtuous person (Annas 2008) or outlined a phenomenology of skill-acquisition where acting ethically is seen as a skill (Dreyfus and Dreyfus 2004). Such studies have contributed with insights as regards the role of moral know-how in moral development. They have not, however, examined bodily dimension of learning to act ethically and becoming virtuous, in any detail.[2] This will be done here. My aim is to examine, phenomenologically, *the role of the body when becoming virtuous* and what *incorporation of virtues-as-skills would mean for perception.* This can further explain the phenomenon of moral perception, contribute to the discussion of alternative approaches to medical ethics and particularly so to the discussion of ethical competence and the *learning of ethics in medical education.*

The text consists of five parts. I start by briefly outlining a virtue ethical approach to medical practice along the lines of Alasdair MacIntyre (1981) and Edmund Pellegrino (1995, 2001).[3] In this reasoning, medicine is seen as a moral practice and an activity through which certain goods, that are internal to the practice, are reached. Virtues are defined in relation to the practice, as learned qualities that promote the achievement of the internal goods of the practice. This enables a discussion of what virtues health care professionals preferably should develop in order for them to achieve the internal goods of medicine. It also opens up a discussion of moral perception in medicine, and the second part contains a short discussion of moral perception and the benefit of seeing virtues-as-skills. The third part turns to phenomenology of the body and presents some core concepts in this perspective. In the fourth part, I examine the role of the body when becoming virtuous and the fifth part examines what it would mean to say that virtues-as-skills should be incorporated, for moral perception in medicine and medical ethics education.

Medicine as a Moral Practice

Medical practice has a scientific side. It is also a moral activity in which decisions are made for the patient's good, based on scientific reasons and the unique patient's situation, her or his goals, preferences and values. Coming from a broadly Aristotelian, teleological framework, some scholars who conceive medicine in this way emphasize that medicine is a practice with a *telos*, an end (Pellegrino 2001, Thomasma 2000). Activities such as curing illness, alleviating pain and suffering, caring, comforting, and helping the patient to cope are all performed in order to achieve this end:

the good health of the patient as a unique person (Pellegrino 2001 pp. 568–569; Pellegrino 1995 p. 267).

This conception of medicine follows Alasdair MacIntyre's (1981) seminal modification of Aristotle's view on practice and virtues, in some important regards. MacIntyre (1981 p. 185) starts by defining practice as a coherent, social activity through which certain goods, which are internal to this practice, are realized. These so-called internal goods cannot be obtained through other means than by those involved in that practice and they can only be specified in terms of that practice. Clinical work qualifies as a practice in this sense, and 'excellence' in curing, alleviating pain, helping others to cope, caring etc. may all be candidates for the label of internal goods.

The benefit of MacIntyre's approach is that it holds together practices, internal goods and virtues. Virtues, in this reasoning, are acquired qualities that enable practitioners to achieve the internal goods. Whereas practitioners may also achieve these goods without virtues, the achievement will be facilitated if they develop the virtues. Virtues, in other words, are defined in relation to the particular practice. The attractiveness of MacIntyre's reasoning may also lie in its simplicity.[4] *If* we could decide how to characterize a particular practice such as that of medicine, we may also be able to describe which goods are internal to this practice and which virtues professionals should develop in order to enable the achievement of these goods.

This is what scholars such as Edmund Pellegrino have sought to do. In his reasoning, the *telos* of medicine as practice is the health of the patient, and 'excellence in healing' is its internal good (Pellegrino 2001 p. 562). Virtues are seen as learnt character traits defined in relation to the practice at stake, as traits 'that dispose its possessor habitually to excellence of intent and performance' as regards the *telos* of medicine (Pellegrino 1995 p. 268). Without virtues, this end would be less optimally attained. Among the candidates for virtues in medical practice, one may find benevolence, compassion and practical wisdom in the sense of *phronesis* (Pellegrino 1995 p. 270). Importantly, however, this reasoning seems to hinge on the idea that medicine is seen a moral practice by its practitioners. If practitioners do not see medicine as a moral practice, they may focus only or primarily on the medical good without noticing the consequences of them failing to see patients as persons in a situational whole.[5] Such practitioners may not notice that the *telos* of medicine hasn't been reached.

This leads to the thorny issue of moral perception. What is it, more precisely, that allows practitioners to see medical practice as a moral activity and an encounter with a patient as a moral situation? Among the various accounts of moral perception, some suggest that any reference to moral perception is only metaphorically meant: any perceptual references need to be scrutinized in detail. Others suggest that moral perception is a perceptual state where we do perceive moral properties of a situation (Audi 2010). Some also turn to a skill model to virtues in order to explain this phenomenon (Jacobson 2006). To this I now turn.

The Skill Model to Virtues and Moral Perception

According to skill models of the virtues, we learn virtues just as skills by practicing them, i.e. through continuous repetition. It takes effort, experience and time. Importantly, the idea is not to conflate virtues with skills, but to explain how virtues are acquired: in ways that are similar to the acquisition of practical skills.

Julia Annas (2008) and Dreyfus and Dreyfus (2004) are useful here. Whereas only Annas is concerned with virtuous becoming, their description of steps in the acquisition of virtues-as-skills (Annas 2008) and acting ethically as a matter of skill (Dreyfus and Dreyfus 2004) share important features. For all of them, the novice typically starts by following certain rules, irrespective of whether the skill in question is driving, acting ethically and/or becoming virtuous. For all of them, acting ethically and/or becoming virtuous is the result of experience, time, effort and habituation. Some features of Dreyfus and Dreyfus's detailed analysis of this are particularly noteworthy.

The novice, Dreyfus and Dreyfus suggest (2004), gains experience by noticing or being told by an instructor to note particularly meaningful aspects of a given situation. After seeing various such situations, subjects will learn to recognize these aspects. Furthermore, as their experience increases, the subjects will come to note more and more meaningful aspects of given situations. This informational abundance needs to be managed, and learners may preferably adopt a coping strategy where they identify a goal that helps them organize the situation in relation to this goal. This allows learners to examine only the smaller set of situational aspects that are relevant for the goal.

Whereas the learner is more competent than the novice at this stage, she or he may still follow a pattern of 'detached planning', involving reflective assessment of features that are salient with respect to the goal, choice of action based on the assessment, which is followed by an emotional experience of the result – such as joy, hope or grief (Dreyfus and Dreyfus 2004 p. 252). In Dreyfus and Dreyfus' account, it takes more experiences of situations of goal-setting, assessment, choice of action and emotionally involved experience of outcome before the learner reaches the stage where she or he is 'struck' by what to do when facing a new though somewhat familiar situation. Yet there is one more step to take for the learner: the step that allows immediate, spontaneous response to a given situation. Even more experiences are needed for the learner to develop a disposition to actions that are likely to result in a desirable outcome. Furthermore, Dreyfus and Dreyfus suggest, as experience of similar situations grows – though they may still require different actions – the subject 'seems gradually to decompose this class of situations into subclasses, each of which shares the same decision, single action, or tactic' (Dreyfus and Dreyfus 2004 p. 253). It is this decomposition that allows an immediate response to the particular situation.

Dreyfus and Dreyfus discuss this as a matter of learning to act ethically, rather than becoming virtuous. Still, I see their reasoning as allowing a more detailed examination also of becoming virtuous. While starting by abiding by rules and noticing or being asked to notice morally relevant features of a certain situation, the learner may gradually come to note many different morally relevant aspects of a given situation (compare Annas 2008). Just as the competent subject of skills, this learner may first need to reflectively assess different situations, deliberate on actions and consider alternative action(s). With more practice, however, this learner may develop a moral competence that allows her or him to see what action is called for in a particular situation – without deliberation.

If we follow the reasoning above, there is nothing mystical about this moral perception. It can be the result of repeated practice that allows the subject gradually to decompose common situations into subclasses, each of which shares the same decision, single action, or tactic *and* to build up a disposition to certain actions. The subject is now able to respond to the situation, in accordance with the acquired virtue-as-skill, in an immediate way. Please note that this is compatible with the view that we sometimes, when facing new ethical situations, will need to deliberate on the appropriateness of how we spontaneously would want to act. Sometimes, we may also fall back on rules and principles in these situations.[6]

Let me now turn to the case of medicine and consider an oft-quoted section from the story *The Death of Ivan Ilych* by Leo Tolstoy. As we enter the story, Ilych has been injured while repairing his newly bought house. To him, this injury is at first not serious, but after a while his situation aggravates. His left side hurts and he has a strange taste in his mouth. He visits a famous doctor in town, but gets deeply frustrated as the doctor ignores his one question 'was his case serious or not?' Tolstoy tells us:

> the doctor ignored that inappropriate question. From his point of view it was not the one under consideration; the real question was to decide between a floating kidney, chronic catarrh, or appendicitis. (Tolstoy 1998 p. 24).

The question, then, is not about Ilych's anxiety, but one of giving an accurate diagnosis. As Ilych is about the leave the doctor's office, he makes one more effort to get an answer to his question: 'We sick people probably often put inappropriate questions. But tell me, in general, is this complaint dangerous, or not …?' (Tolstoy 1998 p. 25). As a response, the doctor looks sternly at him, and states that he has already told him what he considers 'necessary and proper'. The doctor bows, and Ilych leaves the room.[7]

In David J. Casarett's (1999) reading, Ilych's physician seems unable to recognize the moral dimension of medicine, where 'moral' is a synonym for the 'human dimension' of medical practice which includes the patient's fears and worries about illnesses and prognosis (1999 p. 125). The doctor seems to lack the moral perception defined as an ability to recognize the 'moral salience' of a situation.

For Casarett, this perception is a prerequisite for a later moral deliberation on what to do. It can also lead to action without reflective deliberation taking place. One more feature is noteworthy: a failure to *act* may stem from a failure to *see* the moral dimensions of a certain situation. If stated in more positive terms, and in virtue ethical language, the virtuous persons will *see morally relevant features* of a certain situation; they will see *what to do* and – on the basis of their previous evaluations of previous cases and because of them having become virtuous – be *motivated to act* in accordance with what they see (Annas 2004, Nussbaum 1990).

As seen, a virtue-as-skill model can explain how this moral perception can come about. Just as the chess master sees her pawns and the future positional advantages that she may gain on sacrificing one of them, just as the skilled carpenter sees how to build the beautifully winding stairs to the attic while looking at the hole in the ceiling, so will the virtuous person – who has learnt virtue through practice – 'see' what to do in a moral situation. At stake is not some mysteriously perceptible moral properties, but a moral know-how that is learnt through repetition and that feeds into perception.

This clarifies why many medical ethicists within virtue ethical traditions see virtuous becoming as crucial for health care professionals. When having acquired the set of virtues (of relevance for the achievement of the internal goods of medical practice), professionals will more easily see how to act ethically and be motivated to act accordingly. I will henceforward assume that the process of becoming virtuous usefully can be compared to the learning of practical skills.[8] By turning to phenomenology of the body, I hope further to explain how the acquired moral know-how can feed into perception. This also allows an examination of the role of the body in this 'becoming'.

Phenomenology of the Body

The French philosopher Maurice Merleau-Ponty (2006/1945) examines the role of the body for subjective and intersubjective meaning-making. While seeking to overcome the oppositions between the body-as-lived-from-within and the body-as-object, he conceptualizes human existence in terms of the lived body. This concept is meant to denote the body as I live it, in my first-person experiences. The lived body is my lived relationship, as an embodied being, to a world immersed in meaning that I constantly interpret and make meaningful to myself through interaction with others. As Simone de Beauvoir (1949 p. 36, p. 267) puts it, my lived body 'is not a thing, it is a *situation*: it is [my] grasp upon the world and the outline of [my] projects'.

To say that my lived body is my grasp of the world is also to say that I perceive the world from a particular point of view, from my 'now' and 'here', and there is a close linkage between perception, intentionality and orientation in this reasoning. Perception has not only to do with physical sight but also with orientation, i.e. with how we are directed in the world as embodied beings, and with how we are given the world by others. Furthermore, perception immediately and pre-reflectively organizes the world for certain purposes, such as the purpose of engaging with others and the world in an intelligible and successful way.

Now, Merleau-Ponty holds that our basic mode of being is primarily practical and pre-reflective. This mode of existence becomes evident if we consider how the body, in movement, co-ordinates its different parts for the sake of action. When engaging in everyday activities, we are often not reflectively aware of our own locomotion. We seem to act on the basis of a tacit, bodily know-how that has to do with the physical body, a sense of space and of our environment in relation to our bodies. The tacit bodily know-how is what makes it possible for us to engage in various activities without thinking about how to do so.

Merleau-Ponty reconceptualizes the concept of the body schema in order to highlight this bodily know-how that makes the correspondence between embodied subjects and their situations smooth and seamless. The body schema, here, is an implicit, practical awareness of our bodies, motion and space. It is a system of practical and pre-reflective sensory-motor skills that enables action since it makes possible the tacit and seamless co-ordination of different bodily parts in relation to space. Such sensory–motor capabilities may be extended, as when a blind man learns to use a stick. Through repeated motor activity, through habituation, he may come no longer to experience the stick as an object but as an integrated and extended part of her or his lived body (which is not to say that the man experiences the stick as an integrated, extended part of his lived body in exactly the same way as he experiences his hand as an integrated, extended part of his lived body). The stick has, in phenomenological language, become incorporated. The body schema, the subject's system of sensory–motor capabilities, is transformed.

This also matters for the subject's perception. When the stick has become incorporated into the subject's lived body, it opens up new possibilities for the blind man. He can use the stick to reach things that he did not reach before. He finds his way more easily. His transformed body schema allows him to perceive and engage with the world with or through his stick. Furthermore, the blind man no longer needs to attend reflectively to the stick. It is important to note that this receding of the incorporated object from the subject's attention is not accidental. It is crucial.

The receding from reflective awareness can be further explained with Drew Leder's (1990 p. 26) term 'focal disappearance'. The idea is that I cannot at the same time attend *to* my stick as an object of attention and *from* or *through* the stick *to* something else. This helps explain why incorporating the stick is important for the blind man's movement. When incorporated, the stick has become part of that *from* or *through* which the man perceives and engages with the world, and not that *to* which he directs his attention. This is possible precisely because the stick can recede from his reflective awareness. (For further discussion of this, see Zeiler 2012).[9] And, if the blind man should concentrate on the stick itself, i.e. if he should attend thematically and reflectively to the stick and not on where he wants to go, this may disrupt his sense of the space in which he moves. He may risk falling or, at least, bumping into things.

Now, I will suggest that this reasoning also can throw light on the phenomenon of becoming virtuous. It allows an explanation of how repeated practice may transform the subject's lived relation to others and the world, open the world for the subject in certain ways and influence perception – including moral perception as understood in the virtues-as-skills account.

Bodily Becoming: Virtuous

In keeping with his concern with the practical and pre-reflective mode of being, Merleau-Ponty emphasizes that objects in the world do not appear in an allegedly neutral manner to the subject, but through what actions they make possible. In this regard, focus is on intentionality and agency. Furthermore, objects, things and situations also appear in a certain affective mode: as attractive or repulsive, and as inviting us to different responses such as getting closer or withdrawing (Merleau-Ponty 2006. See also Ahmed 2006). In perceiving an object in a particular way, we position ourselves in a certain way towards it or, if one so likes, the object orients us towards it. If we perceive the first tulip in May as beautiful, we may want to get nearer to it; if we perceive a certain situation as calling for moral action, we may feel motivated to such action.

This matters also for the discussion of skill-acquisition. Skills are acquired through our dealings with others, things and situations and they are understood as *acquired dispositions to respond to that which is perceived.* They also form how other human beings, things and situations appear for us in the mode of *calling for response.*

Let me explain this by way of one more example: the person who learns to sail a small sailing boat. As a novice, this person may experience the sea, islands and other boats as intimidating. This can be the case even if the novice has learnt basic navigation rules and the theory of sailing. When on the boat, and while listening to her instructor, the novice may need to focus on her locomotion in relation to the angle of the boat, and particularly so if the boat is small, the wind strong and the novice needs to learn how to lean out of the boat to balance the force of the wind during challenging maneuvers. She needs to think about her locomotion, the strength and angle of the wind and how fast she may want to go, i.e. on how to move the body in relation to the situational whole. Gradually, however, and through repeated practice and habituation, the sailor may come to incorporate the skill of sailing. This being the case, she no longer needs to attend to her own locomotion when engaging in this activity. The skill has become a part of her lived body. To use Leder's formulation above, because the skill can now recede from her reflective awareness, this person need no longer attend to it, but can attend from or through it – as a part of her lived body – to others and to the world –other boats, the sun and the beauty of the surroundings. This may also change the way the sea appears to the subject. It may now present itself as friendly and welcoming rather than scary. When the wind blows, the sea may stand forth to her as calling for a good adventure. It is perceived differently than before.

One of the points with this reasoning is that incorporation of skills opens up the world for the subject in new ways. When incorporated, skills enable action, and recede from the subject's reflective attention. The subject can be 'struck' by what to do and need not think about how to act when acting. This is not to say that an expert sailor 'in the flow' of performance cannot think about future possible moves as a matter of 'reckoning with the possible' (Romdenh-Romluc 2011 p. 100). The point, instead, is that the expert *need* not think about how to sail when engaging in this activity. Furthermore, incorporation can be graded: a skill or object can be more or less deeply or thoroughly incorporated into the subject's lived body. Arguably, the more deeply incorporated it is, the less likely is it that the subject does attend to it (compare Malmqvist and Zeiler 2010, and Zeiler 2012, where the concept of incorporation is applied to beliefs and norms.)

There are, however, reasons to caution against certain ways of discussing incorporation in ethics. What if that which is incorporated into the subject's embodied and habitual engagement with others and the world is not a physical object or skill, but another person? This is what William S. Hamrick (1974 p. 236) suggests in what he calls an ethical example of incorporation, where a parent develops certain habits of caring for her or his child, becomes attuned to the child and its needs, and 'ethically incorporates the child into the way he [or she] habitually inhabits space', What would it mean, more exactly, to incorporate a person? Incorporation has been discussed as the result of repeated motor action and habituation, where that which is incorporated typically recedes from one's reflective attention. However, if that which is incorporated is another person – a subject in my care in the case above – would I then be able to attend to this other person, who is incorporated, while engaging in the activity of caring for her or him? And in activities of care (for the child, for the suffering other) is not one of the crucial ethical that aspects I do attend to this other as a person with her or his own needs, desires and preferences? To say the least, it would be ethically problematic if the other is so deeply incorporated that the subject most often fails to attend to this other as a person in activities of caring for her or him.

One more point is noteworthy. This reasoning highlights the temporal dimension of learning processes and the transformation of lived bodies. Merleau-Ponty sometimes uses the concept of sedimentation in order to emphasize how past experience can feed into, and restrict, our bodily becoming. Sedimentation is the result of us having developed an 'attitude towards the world, when once it has received frequent confirmation, acquires a favoured status for us' (Merleau-Ponty 2006 p. 513). He gives an example: having built our life upon an inferiority complex for many years, it is not easy to change this. As subjects, certain attitudes and patterns of action and being may become our habitual ones, and they will form and inform our style of existence. Importantly for the present reasoning, if someone has built her life upon an inferiority complex, this may also make her *see* certain social situations as intimidating – and she may shy away from such situations without reflectively noticing that she does so. Repeated behaviour over time has resulted in a certain perceptual style. Whereas it takes effort to change such a style – and is perhaps not probable – it is possible and we may through a deliberately chosen alternative behaviour that is repeated over time, change it.

Returning to Medicine

Consider now the medical student who wants to develop virtues that will help her acquire the *telos* of medicine: the good health for the patient as a unique person. On the one hand, she may benefit from taking a course in the philosophy of medicine and medical ethics in order to take time to reflect on different goals of medicine, on ethically difficult but common situations, on what the important virtues, values and ethical principles are in medical practice and how these may underpin or become contradicted by alternative actions; she may also benefit from this in order to learn certain common steps in reflective deliberations in ethically difficult situations. On the other hand, this is hardly enough if someone wants to develop a particular set of virtues. In the virtue-as-skill account, becoming virtuous (and I allow myself not to enter into the discussion of what virtues one may need as a health care professional; as seen above, this has been discussed by others such as Pellegrino 2001) requires experience and repeated practice. Furthermore, I suggest that there is a bodily dimension to this becoming.

Assume that attendance to suffering others as persons is a virtue for medical professionals. If the student wants to develop this virtue, she may start by reflectively thinking about how to do so. She may think about how she approaches patients, what questions she asks, how she listens and, also think about her own and the others' body language. The latter is important since this attentive mode includes much more than linguistic skills. When being self-consciously aware of how she wants to act/be virtuous, she may also reflect on whether she manages to do/be so. In the next step, and in keeping with the phenomenological focus on practice and embodiment, ethical training for health care professionals preferably should not only be theoretical but also practical; it should also, preferably, involve the subject's whole bodily being.

This, I suggest, is the case when Augusto Boal's so-called Moral Agency Theatre is used in medical ethics education. This is a pedagogical method that creates situations characterized by dilemmas, on stage. When presented with the dilemma, some of participants in the Moral Agency Theatre are asked to take on different roles (such as patient and professional) and to try different solutions to the dilemma by improvizing on stage; other participants can volunteer and try other solutions (see Wijma *et al.* 2002 for an example of how moral agency theatre can be used in medical education). The method has the benefit of allowing participants to try different solutions in interaction with others, to feel what it feels like to act in one or the other way, and see how the other person reacts.

This can be one example of how to start to practice ethics in health care, concretely, with one's whole bodily being. This may be a second step – after the theoretical course on philosophy of medicine and medical ethics. Still, however, not even this would be enough for the development of virtues-as-skills, which requires practice over time and habituation. In order to develop the virtue, further repeated action and habituation is needed. This means that whereas virtuous becoming is possible for the medical student witnessing virtuous behaviour in colleagues (where such behaviour includes tone of voice, body posture, tenderness of touching etc.) and take part in for example moral agency education, repeated bodily practice is necessary. This way, the virtue-as-skill of attending to suffering others as persons (or other virtues), may be incorporated into the subject's lived body, and an attending mode of existence may acquire a favoured status for her.

Becoming virtuous takes time and requires practice. Along the way, we may fail to perceive what to do and fail to act even if we see what to do. Still, once a virtue has been incorporated, it can enable ethically skilful engagement with others in medical practice, without the subject having reflectively to deliberate on how to act each time. Instead, this has become a tacit, bodily know-how. And this does not mean that the subject cannot or never will need to reflectively deliberate on what to do. It means that she need not do so in everyday moral situations; instead of focusing on how to be virtuous, she can focus on the patient as a person.[10]

Finally, there is one phenomenological reason why this learning process is particularly important in medicine, if medicine is seen as a moral practice along the lines outlined in the beginning of this chapter (i.e. if it is important that professionals do perceive the moral dimension of this practice). I will now return to the story of Illych to show this.

Illych is worried about his situation, and he is not content with his doctor. Tolstoy does not tell us much about this doctor. In Casarett's reading, however, the doctor lacked moral perception. This failure to see, Casarett suggests, is common today also and it can partly be encouraged by the patients' experiences of illness. Casarett begins with a phenomenological analysis of the experiences of illness. When ill, the subject typically experiences that she cannot engage with others and the world as before. The subject's intentionality is hampered, if not temporarily disrupted. Furthermore, the subject cannot but attend to her or his hurting body-part: her or his attention is drawn to the bodily here and now and more precisely to her or his body part in pain, which the subject may experience as an alien object, as an 'it' (Leder 1990). This alienated relation to one's own body as patient can, Casarett suggests, feed into the professionals' behaviour and turn their attention away from the suffering person as an experiential whole to the body as an object. With a parallel to media, Casarett holds that a 'compelling image has the power to redirect our gaze' and that a similar redirection of attention can take place in medicine.

> Just as the camera and the conjurer draw us in and redirect our gaze, the patient as a subject demands a sympathetic redirection of our gaze toward her/his body. As the patient's body emerges as alien, she finds her attention focused on it, and the gaze of the clinician follows (Casarett 1999 p. 134).

The idea is this: the practitioner's attention is redirected along the lines of the patient's own attention, to the hurting body part, to the body as an object.

On the one hand, the doctor – when following the patient's attention – will focus on the body part in pain and this is of course important. On the other hand, if this becomes the only loci of attention, the patient's whole bodily situation including her or his fears, worries, preferences and goals may recede from the physician's attention. And this can be unfortunate in cases where the patients' whole situation requires attention – as in many ethically difficult situations where it is unclear what it best for this particular patient.

Casarett suggests that lack of sensitivity on the part of Ilych's doctor and possibly others may be due to the way we, when in pain, focus on experiences of pain in a way that direct clinicians' attention to the body as an object. If Casarett's reasoning is right in this – and I think he has a point – it becomes all the more important for medical professionals to learn a certain kind of attention to suffering others to the extent that it becomes a disposition to certain action that function on a pre-reflective level. I see such an attentive mode of being as a virtue. And in the skill model to virtues, it takes time, experience and effort to acquire such a virtue. Still, if practitioners otherwise may follow the attention of their patients, this virtue-as-skill would benefit from being repeated until it is incorporated.

Part Two

When High-Tech Medicine Fails: Old Age, Dying and Mental Illness

Chapter 4

Old Age and Dependency

Eric Matthews

Introduction

Old age cannot be defined simply in terms of the number of years someone has been alive: as the normal life-span has extended, so the age at which we perceive someone as 'old' has changed. It should rather be thought of as the final phase of life. It is common to see a human life as consisting of successive stages, as in Shakespeare's familiar lines about the seven ages of a man in Act 2, Scene 7 of *As You Like It.* The distinct scenes in the drama of a life are outlined, starting with infancy and culminating in the final scene, of 'second childishness and mere oblivion, sans teeth, sans eyes, sans taste, sans everything'. As Shakespeare's words imply, we traditionally conceive of old age, not simply as the end phase of life, but also as a period of *decline.* Aging is the time of increasing frailty, physical and mental – a slowing of mental activity and loss of memory, together with impaired physical mobility and an increased liability to certain distressing and disabling diseases, such as cancer, Type 2 diabetes, and arthritis. All these together mean decreased ability to look after oneself and one's needs. Shakespeare's phrase 'second childishness' is significant, since in some ways, to age is to return to the vulnerability and helplessness of infancy.

Of course, not all old people are as decrepit as Shakespeare's description would suggest: it has always been true that many old people have been fit and active, and the proportion has increased as a result of medical progress and improved living conditions. Some even predict a future 'end of aging', as a result of scientific developments. If they are right, this will create different kinds of ethical and philosophical problems. But there seems little immediate prospect of this coming about: for the foreseeable future, we are confronted by the ethical questions which arise from the increasing *dependency* of human beings in old age.

There is one particular disease to which older people are more liable than younger (though it can also have an earlier onset) which can be seen as embodying the helplessness of old age in its most extreme form. This is dementia, of which the best-known type is perhaps Alzheimer's Disease. The ethical problems raised by dementia likewise seem to be extreme versions of those which face us when we reflect on the care and treatment of old people generally. But we need to be careful here. Dementia, in its most severe manifestations, results in a loss of physical and especially mental capacities that is *so* extreme that it is not illuminating to compare it with the dependency of what we can call 'normal' old age. For this reason, I shall in this chapter mainly treat the ethical problems of dementia separately from those of aging in general.

The association of old age with increasing frailty and loss of mental capacity is liable to colour the experience which many old people have of dealings with their doctors and other health care professionals. They may, for example, have to put up with doctors and nurses talking about them, in their presence, in the third person, as if they were incapable of participating in the discussion. Similarly, they may find doctors asking their *carers* questions about their wishes or needs (e.g. 'What are her symptoms?' or 'Where does she feel the pain?'), rather than directing their questions to the patients themselves. If they are addressed directly, it may well be in over-simplified language, of the kind one might use in speaking to a very small child. Again, as Wicclair (1993 p. 121) says, doctors, nurses and social workers may sometimes withhold essential information about the patient's condition from older people in order to 'protect' them, or 'for their own good'. Ahronheim *et al.* (1994 p. 56) say that there is still a tendency in some places 'to regard advanced age as automatically disqualifying a patient from being told the truth about his or her condition'.

The prevalence of this tendency should not be exaggerated: it is far from being a universal feature of old people's experience. But it is not uncommon, and when it does occur it represents a literally paternalistic attitude. Old people in these cases are indeed treated like small children (Shakespeare's 'second childishness' again), who are incapable of participating in normal adult relationships. But, whereas it may be acceptable to deal with small children in this way, it shows a lack of respect to do so with people who can draw upon a lifetime's experience of such relationships. I shall consider the issues which this raises in a later section.

Is Autonomy the Central Issue?

Many discussions of the ethics of treating older patients in the current literature start from what is supposed to be a Kantian perspective on ethics, though it is, I shall argue, a misinterpretation of Kant. For Kant, the essence of ethics is respect for persons, where being a person is defined in terms of 'autonomy', which literally means 'self-government'. Kantian persons are said to 'legislate' for themselves, like an autonomous state. Onora O'Neill says, 'he [Kant] does not equate it [autonomy] with any distinctive form of personal independence or self-expression, let alone with acting on some rather than other sorts of preferences.' (O'Neill 2002 p. 83). Persons 'legislate for themselves' only in the sense that they act on principles which are approved by reason, a capacity which they share with other persons, not by emotions or interests which are peculiar to them as individuals. As O'Neill goes on, 'Kantian autonomy is manifested in a life in which duties are met, in which there is respect for others and their rights, rather than in a life liberated from all bonds.' (O'Neill 2002 p. 83).

It is because of this that Kant sees autonomy as 'the ground of the dignity of human nature and of every rational nature' (Kant 1998 p. 43). Persons are worthy of moral respect because they possess reason, the capacity to assess principles of action, not in terms of whether they satisfy purely personal needs or desires, but in terms of their suitability to be laws governing the dealings of any mutually respectful beings with each other.

In modern liberal medical ethics, the principle of respect for patient autonomy has assumed fundamental importance. As O'Neill says, since the 1970s 'the importance of respecting individual rights and individual autonomy' has become 'the dominant ethical idea in many discussions of topics ranging from genetic testing to geriatric medicine' (O'Neill 2002 p. 2). If asked for a philosophical justification of the importance of autonomy, most ethicists would probably do so in Kantian terms – that it is our possession of autonomy which makes us worthy of moral respect. But there is a subtle, but important, difference between the modern conception of autonomy and Kant's. Above all, the modern conception is one of *individual* autonomy, and that affects the meaning of 'rationality'. For Kant, reason was our means of recognizing objective and absolute moral principles, which were the same for all rational beings. In modern liberal thought, however, reason is our means of arriving, by reflection on our own experience, at *our own* values – the values by which *we* wish to live our lives, which may not be those which other, equally rational, beings would recognize.

In the modern conception, autonomy is to be valued, as Ronald Dworkin says, because it protects 'the capacity to express one's own character – values, commitments, convictions, and ... interests' (Dworkin 1993 p. 224). In this interpretation, as Dworkin also says, the basis for respect for autonomy is a recognition of the right to make one's own decisions even when they might be regarded by others (and even perhaps by oneself) as *ir*rational. To be autonomous is to be capable of taking independent control of one's life. In medical contexts, this means that autonomy is exhibited above all in deciding to accept or refuse treatment, and respect for patient autonomy comes to mean mainly an insistence on *informed consent* to treatment. The patient alone must decide, on the basis of his or her own values, and in the light of full information about the nature and consequences of the proposed treatment, whether to accept or reject it. This in turn implies that the autonomous patient has a right to be told the truth about his or her condition. Since no one else can make decisions about treatment on the patient's behalf, it might also be held to imply a right to confidentiality – that is, the right that information about the patient's condition should not be disclosed, without the patient's consent, to anyone other than those who need to know it if they are to give appropriate treatment.

But the ageist stereotypes of old people create a difficulty for ethical discussions at this point. If respect for patient autonomy (and so for the human dignity of patients) is respect for their capacity to make independent treatment decisions; and if old age is essentially a period of progressive decline in capacities (including this one), then how do we respect the human dignity of older people? Do people as they age become increasingly less than full, adult, persons, and more like children, who can only be treated paternalistically, that is, have to have treatment decisions made for them by others who know better what is good for the patient? Is it relevant, from this point of view, that, as Malcolm Bavidge reminds us, 'losing one's competence and personality after a long life is a very different prospect from the incompetence that characterizes the infant' (Bavidge, in Hughes *et al.* 2006 p. 47).

These questions are at the heart of much of the recent discussion in the literature of the ethics of caring for older people. Some writers try to deal with them by speaking of 'partial autonomy' (e.g. Martin Vernon, in Rai (ed.) 2004 p. 23). That is, a decline in competence with age is seen as a decline from the *full* autonomy of earlier adult years to an autonomy which is progressively more limited in scope, which can be appealed to in some cases but not in others. In the same vein, Feinberg argues that autonomy should be considered as what he calls a 'variable concept', 'with higher and lower cut-off points depending on the nature of the circumstances, the interests at stake, and the moral or legal purposes to be served' (Feinberg 1986 p. 117). For example, 'The more risky the conduct, the greater the degree of voluntariness required'. Such proposals, unlike Kant, treat autonomy, not as an all-or-nothing concept, but as something which can exist to a greater or lesser degree. Some would then lay an ethical duty on carers to make every effort to establish the degree of competency which the old person retains. Since the very conditions in which the old person is being cared for may encourage an attitude of dependence, a feeling on the part of the person herself of incompetence to make decisions, Buchanan and Brock suggest that 'Reasonable efforts must be made to restore or enhance competence where possible' (Buchanan and Brock 1989 p. 285). It is arguable that this implies that there is an ethical obligation to provide resources for improving the physical environment in which care is given. Creating a brighter and more personalized setting (for instance with more of the patient's personal possessions), and providing activities which maintain some continuity with the patient's past life can reinforce their sense of individual identity.

Other discussions in the literature have concerned the alleged problems of communicating with older patients about their condition. Wicclair (1993 p. 121) describes how doctors, nurses and social workers (and, he might also have added, relatives) may sometimes withhold information from elderly patients 'for their own good'. An example of this is cited by Ahronheim *et al.* (Ahronheim *et al.* 1994 p. 117). An eighty-year old woman (whom they call 'Lilian') suffered from dysphagia (difficulty in eating), which a biopsy revealed to be due to cancer. There was no way to avoid this eventually becoming a total obstruction, but immediate and drastic surgery would at least postpone the development of this obstruction. But her son asked the doctors not to reveal the diagnosis to his mother, on the grounds that she would not 'tolerate' it, or the disfiguring operation which they proposed. For much the same reason, as Martin Vernon writes (in Rai 2004 p. 10) doctors may find it simpler to talk to the relatives of very frail old people. The ethical issue which such practices raise is whether doctors and other carers are right to yield to this temptation. The answer seems to be that it is quite wrong to infer, from physical dependence, a lack of competence to make independent decisions, for example, about treatment – as wrong in the case of older people as it would be at any age. If so, then a frail old person has as much right as anyone to be given the full information, however unpleasant it may be, which she needs to make a free decision to accept or refuse treatment. Any difficulty which patients may have in 'tolerating' information can often be lessened, in this case as in others, by finding gentler ways of breaking bad news.

Autonomy and Dementia

Questions about autonomy and paternalism are less easily dealt with when the decline in mental capacity associated with aging has progressed further, and in particular in cases of severe dementia. On Dworkin's interpretation of the moral basis for respecting autonomy, to exercise autonomy one must have some conception of a continuing self, and this is precisely what one loses as aging and above all dementia progressively destroys memory, and so continuity with one's past life. A severely demented person no longer has much consciousness of herself as an individual, with 'values, commitments, convictions' of her own (Dworkin 1993 p. 224). Dementia is a slowly developing disease, and in its earlier stages, the person still retains some elements of her earlier individual self – some sense of who she is, some memories of her past, a recognition of significant others and so the basis for a continuing relationship with them. She also remains competent to make at least some decisions about her treatment 'at least at certain times, in certain environments' (Buchanan and Brock 1989 p. 281). In the earlier stages of dementia, therefore, we can ascribe Feinberg's 'partial autonomy' to patients, so that no special ethical difficulties about respecting autonomy need arise.

But, as the disease progresses, these remaining elements of 'selfhood' disappear. The person loses all ability to recognize others, even those closest to her, and eventually may lose even a sense of who she herself is. In that case, Dworkin asks, 'Should we care about the dignity of a dementia patient if he himself has no sense of it?' (Dworkin 1993 p. 221). For Dworkin, as for many other writers, respect for dignity is primarily respect for the right to make decisions for oneself, especially when those decisions do not seem to others to be in the patient's own interests. He cites the example of a woman he calls 'Mary', who could not recognize relatives and had forgotten how to manage a bath tub. Should she, he asks, 'be allowed to spend or give away her money as she wishes, or to refuse prescribed medical treatment, or to decide which relative is appointed as her guardian? Should she be allowed to insist that she be cared for at home, in spite of her family's opinion that she would get better care in an institution?' (*ibid.* p. 222).

As Dworkin suggests, one way to deal with the general question of respect for the dignity of a severely demented person is to remember the dignity which she *used* to have, in the course of her whole life so far: she may not now be a 'person' in the fullest sense, but she should be respected because she *has been* one (*ibid.* p. 221). This is the position taken also by Campbell *et al.*, who say, 'The dignity they once had and elicited undergirds how they are to be treated in the present' (Campbell *et al.* 2005 p. 199). But this clearly will not, in itself, resolve the problems about making treatment decisions. These decisions need to be made *in the present*, and in the present the severely demented patient lacks all capacity to make them – no sense of who she is, and so what her best interests might be, and no ability to foresee how those interests might best be served in the future. One answer considered by Dworkin is that, at least in this stage of dementia, the patient's right to be treated beneficently trumps the right to make autonomous decisions (since she has no capacity to make such decisions, anyway). The person with advanced dementia 'still has the right to beneficence, the right that decisions on these matters be made in his best interests ... But he no longer has the right, as competent people do, himself to decide contrary to these interests' (Dworkin 1993 p. 225). But, at best, this seems to put severely demented old people in the same position from an ethical point of view as very small children, ignoring the differences already mentioned between infants and old people, however incompetent they may now be. Surely, one might feel, an adequate ethics ought to be able to accommodate that distinction.

It is presumably for this reason that Dworkin and others suggest that their earlier exercise of autonomy could be used to make up for their lack of autonomy in the present. They may, for example, have made an advance directive when they were still competent. This may take the form of a 'living will', a written, signed and witnessed, document stating the kinds of treatment that, at the time when they made the will, they wanted, or, more usually, did *not* want, to be given in particular future circumstances (e.g. in the event of their becoming incompetent). Or, again when still competent, they may have appointed someone else to make decisions on their behalf for when they themselves were no longer able to do so. The proxy decision-maker would be someone on whom they felt they could rely to make the kind of decisions which they themselves would have made in the circumstances, if they had been able to.

But there are problems with all these methods of substituted decision-making. One practical difficulty is that, at present, relatively few people draw up living wills, or appoint proxy decision-makers. This could, perhaps, be alleviated by programmes of publicity aimed at promoting the practice of making advance directives. But objections of principle have also been made. Buchanan and Brock, for instance, argue that 'they [living wills] are too general and vague to provide clear guidance on decisions to forgo life-sustaining treatment or care' (Buchanan and Brock 1989 p. 296). At the time when someone makes a living will, or appoints a proxy decision-maker, they cannot possibly predict the *exact* circumstances in which the relevant future decisions will have to be made, but these circumstances are often as important as any general principle in determining what it is best to do. A younger person may well feel, for example, that they do not wish to be kept alive if they become demented. But if, say, they could know that they would still be in reasonably comfortable circumstances, with attentive carers, that might affect their decision. A proxy decision-maker is, of course, in a better position to know the particular circumstances which prevail at the time when the decision has to be made. But it is risky to assume that the proxy knows the patient's mind well enough to be able to interpret how the patient would have decided in these circumstances, if she had been competent to make a decision. And there is an even more fundamental objection of principle. Relying on advance directives depends on the assumption that the values which someone had in the past will necessarily be those which he or she has now. But even in normal circumstances our values and preferences change and develop, in line with the changes in our lives and our reflections on those changes. In the case of a person with severe dementia, we must take account, in addition, of the radical discontinuity in someone's life resulting from the dementia itself – the disruption of personal memories and of one's former relationships with significant others. If one wants to hold on to the view that respect for individual autonomy, in the sense of decision-making competence, is important to respect for human dignity, then it may be that reliance on advance directives is the nearest one can get to affirming the human dignity of severely demented people. But perhaps that should lead us to question this conception of autonomy and its ethical centrality.

The Ethical Importance of Dependency

There are two questions to be considered here: should we conceive of respect for autonomy as consisting only in respect for treatment decisions made by fully competent adults, in possession of all relevant information? And, does the respect for human dignity, which must be the heart of any ethics worthy of the name, consist only in respect for autonomy in this sense? One philosopher who has argued for a re-examination of the concept of autonomy, especially in the context of care of the elderly, is George Agich (see, for example, Agich 2003 p. 6–7 and 2007 p. 73–4). He argues that the meaning of 'autonomy' must be context-dependent: the wide range of use of the term in the bioethics literature on care of the aged suggests, he says, 'that it is unlikely that an essential or core meaning underlies these various employments' (Agich 2003 p. 6). Nevertheless, he goes on, we cannot ignore the *cultural* significance of the idea of autonomy, especially in American society. It is a cultural ideal in American (and, one might add, more widely in Western) society that personhood is expressed in independence and self-reliance – the ability to make one's own decisions about one's life, on the basis of one's own values. But the characteristic feature of aging people, especially of those in long-term care who are the main focus of Agich's discussion, is precisely *dependence*. 'The challenging question', Agich says, 'is how can considerations of autonomy apply to these situations and, of equal importance, what practical guidance can the appeal to autonomy provide for these elusive situations' (Agich 2007 p. 74). The process of aging involves a progressive diminution of one's self-reliance and so an increasing dependence on carers. The relation of old people to carers is therefore not that between two sovereign individuals, as presupposed in the standard modern bioethical conception of autonomy. But neither, Agich argues, is it like that between a parent and a small child, as embodied in the concept of 'paternalism'. It cannot be like that, Agich contends, because the identity and sense of self of an adult are far more developed than those of a small child. 'Hence, the mutuality of the care giving relationship with dependent adults occurs at more complex levels of communication that are not analogous to the paradigmatic mother–infant relationship and not reducible to affective states akin to maternal affection' (*ibid.* p. 83). Emphasis on the model of autonomy as independence makes it look as if all ethical issues in the care of the aged were problems about the defence of the rights of patients to shape their own lives against medical paternalism. These problems are then thought to be dealt with 'by establishing legal rights or promulgating regulations', in order to 'force caregivers to conform to the standards of a liberal polity and respect the rights of their wards' (Agich 2003 p. 11).

The formulation of an alternative account of autonomy, as Agich sees, requires a philosophical re-examination of the concept of a person. The Kantian concept of autonomy, and its modern bioethical derivatives, presupposes a Cartesian dualism which makes a distinction between being a 'person' and being a 'human being'. For Descartes, what I essentially am is 'a thing that thinks', where a 'thinking' thing is 'a thing that doubts, affirms, denies, understands a few things, is ignorant of many things, is willing, is unwilling, and also which imagines and has sensory perceptions' (Descartes 1988 p. 87). Being a 'self' or 'person', in other words, is defined entirely in terms of thought (even the sensory perceptions and imagination referred to are included in the definition only insofar as they are 'modes of thinking'). And to be a mode of thinking is to exist 'within me' (*ibid.*). What constitutes me as a person, and so, in Kantian ethics, as worthy of moral respect, is thus entirely a matter of what goes on inside me, independently of any relation to the outside world, including other people. Specifically, it is a matter of the operations of my reasoning, or cognitive, powers. The human beings that we actually encounter, however, in caring for them, for instance, are much more than their inner selves, or their cognitive and conative capacities. They also have emotions and bodily needs, and relations to other people. Even our most intellectual thoughts are not independent of either our emotions or our relations to other people. A failure to understand our dependence on others, as Alasdair MacIntyre argues, 'is apt to obscure some features of rational agency' (MacIntyre 1999 p. 8). This is because we have to interact with others in ways which involve 'responsive sympathy and empathy' if we are to understand what constitutes rationality in acting, and so to make their actions intelligible to us, and ours in turn to them (*ibid.* p. 14).

In this sense, the Cartesian (and Kantian) conception of a person, as a kind of disembodied and disinterested thinker and decision-maker, is of an abstraction from the whole human being. It is the product of an analytic approach to philosophy, which conceives of its task as a purely *a priori* 'conceptual analysis', without taking due account of our concrete experience of the world, from which these concepts are derived. What we need, as Agich suggests, is a more *phenomenological* account, that is, one which, in Husserl's words, gets 'back to the things themselves', as we actually experience them. What this means in this case is setting aside conceptions of personhood arrived at by metaphysical argument (as Descartes's was as a by-product of a search for indubitable foundations of knowledge), in favour of reflection on human beings as we actually encounter them. If the concept of a 'person' is to have any meaning for us, it must be derived from our experience of our fellow human beings. That experience takes the form, in the first instance, of *communicating* with them, not only by the use of language, but by means of our mutual *responses* to each other, emotional and even sensual. It is this communication, in all its complexity, which distinguishes someone as a 'person', rather than a mere 'object', which can be considered purely from the outside. It differentiates persons also from non-human animals, with which we can have much more limited communication, just because they are not of our species and so do not respond to us in characteristically *human* ways. Even small children can take part in this human communication, though of course in a simpler and less developed way than adults. In the mutuality of our responses, we recognize someone else as a being like ourselves, a separate subject of experience, worthy of the same respect that we demand for ourselves. As Tom Kitwood says, '[Personhood] is a standing or status that is bestowed upon one human being by others, in the context of relationship and social being. It implies recognition, respect and trust' (Kitwood 1997 p. 8).

This is the conception of a human being developed by such phenomenologists as Heidegger and Merleau-Ponty. Both argue that our mode of existence, as human beings, is 'being-in-the-world'. Heidegger explains what he means by this (Heidegger 1962 p. 95): '... our everyday Being-in-the-world, which we also call our '*dealings*' *in* the world and *with* entities within the world. Such dealings have already dispersed themselves into manifold ways of concern' (Heidegger's italics). In other words, our humanity is to be found, not in our possession of a purely interior 'self', but in our ways of relating to the world of objects and people around us. These relationships, furthermore, are not purely theoretical or intellectual, but involve the practical and emotional *meaning* which objects and people have for us, and which we share with other human beings.

Merleau-Ponty takes up this view of the human mode of being, and develops, as a fundamental theme of his philosophy, its implication – that human beings are essentially *embodied*. Unless we were embodied, we could not have our being 'in-the-world': our bodies give us a place in the world, among objects, from which we can have an individual perspective on the world. But our bodies are not in the world simply as objects, with purely spatial and causal relationships to other objects. Our ability to communicate with each other entails that we are embodied *subjects*, beings for whom our surrounding world is *meaningful*: our relation to the objects around us is, to use Heidegger's words, that we have 'dealings' with it and 'concerns' about it. These dealings and concerns are not only (indeed, not mostly) very high-flown. Just because we are embodied, we interact with the world at many levels, from the deeply personal to the more or less impersonal. In ways like this, our embodiment is the source of our most basic engagement with the world, from which our fully conscious and rational personhood emerges, and even then only sporadically. As Merleau-Ponty puts it: 'Thus there appears round our personal existence a margin of *almost* impersonal existence', so that 'Personal existence is intermittent' (Merleau-Ponty 2006 p. 84).

My identity as an individual, on this view, goes beyond the conscious sense of myself. It develops in the course of my life, as experiences accumulate, and are remembered. These memories are themselves not necessarily conscious, but are 'sedimented' (to use Merleau-Ponty's term) in my bodily habits of response, so that they continue to constitute an individual identity even when conscious recollection is lost. The significance of this in the present context is that it implies that the humanity which is worthy of moral respect, of being treated, in Kant's words, as an 'end-in-itself' and never simply as a means, is located not only in our rational capacities, but in all levels of our being as embodied human subjects. This is not to say that our rational capacities, such as our capacity to make explicit decisions about treatment or non-treatment, are not important parts of our humanity, indeed the fullest development of what makes us human. Those who are demented have undoubtedly lost something: the point is that they have not lost *everything* which is worthy of moral respect. They remain subjects, able to communicate with other subjects and so to be recognized by them as separate individuals.

To the extent that people of any age possess the capacity to make treatment-decisions for themselves, respect for their humanity requires doctors and other carers to respect those decisions. But respect for the right of competent patients to make their own treatment decisions is not the only way in which we need to respect humanity. We need to recognize, as Alasdair MacIntyre argues, that 'human vulnerability, and our consequent dependence on others' (MacIntyre 1999 p. 1) are as much deserving of moral concern as our rationality. All the forms of infantilization referred to earlier are morally unacceptable. More positively, every effort must be made to cherish what remains of their individual identity. Concern for humanity is shown as much by such simple gestures as taking time to talk to them as fellow adults and by finding ways of prompting recollection of their past lives as by seeking consent to treatment.

Nevertheless, there are implications for the choice of treatment. Even if a very frail elderly patient is unable to communicate verbally, or sign a consent form, she remains a person, a human being with wishes and preferences about treatment which deserve respect. These preferences may still be communicable in non-verbal ways, and there is a moral duty on those caring for her to develop the skills required to decipher these communications. As George Agich says, perhaps we should 'understand consent as a process that permeates the care-giving relationship … [which] requires a continuous dialogue between health professionals and patients' (Agich 1993 p. 83). The time required for this process may simply be unavailable in the case of those dramatic treatment decisions which tend to preoccupy the ethical literature. But, as Agich says, much of the care of the elderly is long-term, in which talk of discrete 'treatments' is hardly realistic. In their relationship with their carers, old people can establish their identity, and so their preferences, sufficiently clearly to show, in broad terms at least, how they wish to be treated. Such wishes need to be taken into account, even if they are not ultimately determinant of the decision about treatment.

In severe dementia, these relationships will probably be impoverished: they will not, for instance, include a patient's reminiscence about her own past. But the patient remains a person even so, on the account of personhood given above. Even if she lacks a conscious sense of self, her humanity and individuality are still shown in her capacity to respond in human and individual ways to others. This individual identity, because sedimented by a lifetime of experience, is much more complex than that of a child. Hence, it is still ethically important to avoid any form of infantilizing treatment. In short, the central contention of this chapter is that the excessively rational conception of personhood which underlies much recent literature in medical ethics is both philosophically misguided and inadequate to dealing with the moral problems which arise in caring for those whose very vulnerability most demands concern for their human worth.

Chapter 5

An Ethical Enquiry into the Concept of Palliative Care

Rien MJPA Janssens and Guy AM Widdershoven

Introduction

Palliative care is a relatively new phenomenon in many European health care systems. Its origins are mostly traced back to 1967, when Cicely Saunders founded the first modern hospice in London: St Christopher's Hospice. Only during the last quarter of the twentieth century has palliative care attracted attention in other European countries as well as in North America. But since then, developments have been rapid. Palliative care in the early twenty-first century is in many countries at the focus of attention. Not only are the type and number of institutions increasing in many countries, but the concept of palliative care is also changing, new definitions have been proposed and the ethical dilemmas in palliative care are still vehemently discussed within different cultural contexts. While the origins of palliative care can be found in the hospice movement, palliative care is now being organized in a variety of settings, inside and outside the health care system. Cancer care is no longer the exclusive domain of palliative care and the variety of patients receiving palliative care is also increasing. And while hospice care used to be associated with terminal care, the consensus now is that the provision of palliative care can go hand in hand with curative or life-prolonging treatment. Palliative care, it is argued, starts from the time of diagnosis, or even earlier. Setting, time path and type of care are all under change with significant consequences for the concept of palliative care.

In this chapter, we will investigate these developments in palliative care. For a critical comprehension of palliative care in the beginning of the twenty-first century, it is imperative to examine the historical development of palliative care. What were the initial motivations of the young hospice movement and what can these motivations tell us about the moral significance of palliative care now? Is hospice, conceived as a philosophy or ideology of care, still of influence in the current ethical debates on decision-making at the end of life? Or are new forces at work that have decreased the significance of traditional hospice values? Based on this historical analysis of hospice values (Section 1), we will explain in Section 2 how values in modern palliative care have developed. While modern palliative care was influenced by the hospice movement, the new settings in which it became organized were also influential. We will argue in Section 3 that the modern concept of palliative care has become ambiguous. The practice of palliative care is difficult to demarcate from other practices and its values and norms regarding end-of-life decision-making are increasingly under debate. In the fourth section, we will argue that the concept of palliative care is in need of new critical reappraisal. Moreover, we propose that a critical analysis of the values underpinning palliative care requires input from hermeneutic ethics. Indeed, hermeneutic ethics can help improve normative debates on moral dilemmas in palliative care.

Historical Overview of Hospice and Terminal Care

The earliest hospices were established in the early Christian era. These were guest houses for pilgrims and other travellers where care was provided in order to enable the guests to continue their pilgrimages. Caregivers were inspired by the gospels, especially the seven works of grace mentioned in the gospel of St. Matthew. In 1842, the term 'hospice' was for the first time associated with care for the dying as Mme Jeanne Garnier formed the 'Association des Dames du Calvaire' and opened a home for the dying a year later (Clark 2000). In 1879, the Sisters of Charity founded Our Lady's Hospice for the Dying in Dublin. Medical and nursing care were not well developed and the focus of care was on what the Sisters called 'soul-cures'. Historical research has revealed that pain and symptom treatment were primarily instrumental to the higher goal of spiritual reconciliation, or if necessary of religious conversion, of poor patients who had turned away from the church (Humphreys 2000; Humphreys 2001). Around the turn of the century, several hospices were established in the UK. Already in the beginning of the 1950s, Saunders observed the regular giving of morphine in St Luke's hospice, a method of treating pain she later introduced in St Joseph's. As early as 1960, she writes: 'Constant pain needs constant control' (Saunders 1960a p. 17, quoted in Clark 1999). Patients should not have to ask for pain relief. Rather, in order to help patients maintain their independence, regular drugs is the cardinal rule. Saunders has always stressed the importance of anticipation in terminal care.

It was also in these older hospices where Cicely Saunders developed her ideas about truth-telling. She criticized common practice at that time where patients were deliberately deceived, and she opted for a more individual approach, depending on what the patient wanted to know. With regard to truth-telling, she writes in 1965: 'In this, as in many other things, we cannot hurry the dying but we must let them teach us' (Saunders 1965a, quoted in Clark 1999). While not advocating truth-telling at all times, she is sensitive to the distress that may be caused by withholding information to the patient.

While patients dying from cancer were still largely overlooked within the mainstream health care systems, concerns about the medical neglect of cancer patients slowly started to increase. The first pain clinics originated in the 1950s, progress was made in the area of (palliative) radiotherapy and chemotherapy, and attention was drawn to the psychosocial needs of cancer patients and their loved ones. Elisabeth Kübler-Ross spoke with dying patients in American hospitals and based on this work she published her bestseller in 1969 (Kübler-Ross 1969). She observed in her patients five different phases characteristic of the emotional situations they were in: denial, anger, bargaining, depression and acceptance. Although she acknowledged that all emotions should be allowed to exist, a goal of psychosocial care was to help patients accept their finiteness.

St Christopher's hospice, the first modern hospice with research and teaching facilities, was founded as a reaction to the care for the dying in general hospitals. According to Saunders: 'the last stages of life should not be seen as defeat, but rather as life's fulfilment' (Saunders 1965b). The tertiary NHS hospitals with their curative focus were ill equipped to provide management of terminally ill patients. A new concept of care was to originate outside the institutions of the formal health care system.

In the context of an increasing technologically driven medicine, not only did the hospice movement flourish, but so did membership of the British Voluntary Euthanasia Society. In 1969, a Voluntary Euthanasia bill was discussed and rejected in the House of Lords. The young hospice movement was characterized by a strong moral discomfort with voices in the UK pleading for the legalization of euthanasia.The arguments of the hospice movement against euthanasia were mainly religious in character. Even in the very terminal stages of illness, patients can find reconciliation. Since reconciliation is considered to be God's gift of grace, and not for man to decide, ending the life of a patient prematurely may well keep the patient from receiving God's grace.

Originally hospice was not associated with palliation. According to Saunders, the terminal stage begins when 'all curative and palliative measures have been exhausted' (Saunders 1960a p. 16). In 1966, she defines terminal illness as 'a claim for comfort rather than curative or even palliative procedures' (Saunders 1966 p. 225). Treatable patients can be palliated whereas terminal patients require comfort care only.

The Origins of Modern Palliative Care

Saunders' publications became well-known in Canada and the USA where psychosocial care for the dying had already gained impetus due to the work of Kübler-Ross. In 1975, Balfour Mount founded the first palliative care unit in Montreal, Canada. Because the term 'hospice' in Latin languages, including French, has negative associations, denoting an institution for the destitute, Balfour Mount coined the term palliative care as a translation of hospice care, or terminal care. From this time on, palliative care started to be re-integrated into the health care systems as was initially foreseen and hoped for by Saunders. Palliative care was to become implemented in a variety of settings, ranging from home care to the acute hospital care. Thus, palliative care, in contrast to hospice care, began in the tertiary hospital setting (Gracia 2002).

In 1987, palliative medicine was recognized in the UK as a subspecialty of general medicine and later as an official medical specialty (Doyle *et al.* 1996). In 2002, Palliative care was defined by the World Health Organization as follows:

> Palliative care is an approach that improves the quality of life of patients and their families facing the problems associated with life-threatening illness, through the prevention and relief of suffering by means of early identification and impeccable assessment and treatment of pain and other problems, physical, psychosocial and spiritual. Palliative care:
>
> - provides relief from pain and other distressing symptoms
> - affirms life and regards dying as a normal process
> - intends neither to hasten nor postpone death
> - integrates the psychological and spiritual aspects of patient care

- offers a support system to help patients live as actively as possible until death
- offers a support system to help the family cope during the patient's illness and in their own bereavement
- uses a team approach to address the needs of patients and their families, including bereavement counselling, if indicated
- will enhance quality of life, and may also positively influence the course of illness
- is applicable early in the course of illness, in conjunction with other therapies that are intended to prolong life, such as chemotherapy or radiation therapy, and includes those investigations needed to better understand and manage distressing clinical complications (WHO 2002).

Noteworthy in this definition, and contrary to an earlier definition of 1990, there is no mention of a pathology (the older definition contained the term 'cancer'). Furthermore, palliative care is described as an approach that improves the quality of life of patients *and* families. Such an approach can be applied to almost all medical specialties. It does not help demarcate palliative care from other forms of care. Moreover, palliative care is meant for patients with life-threatening illness, although this does not necessarily mean they are going to die. This is corroborated by the last statement that palliative care can go hand in hand with life prolongation. However, it is also stated that palliative care should not strive to postpone death. If that is so, palliative care would exclude curative actions or even life-prolongation. The definition appears to be ambiguous with regard to the scope of palliative care. A last striking point to be made is that the definition explicitly rejects euthanasia, at least within the domain of palliative care: palliative care does not intend to hasten death. In this respect, the hospice values are still influential in modern palliative care.

The definition thus denotes important characteristics of palliative care, reminiscent of the hospice tradition from which it originates. Prevention and early identification for instance were already central in Cicely Saunders' thinking before the opening of St Christopher's. The idea that medical care is only one realm within palliative care, next to psychosocial and spiritual care, is as old as the earliest hospices for the dying (spiritual care was at the heart of the older hospices). The idea that dying is a normal process was present in the early writings of Cicely Saunders. In 1960, she compares life to a pilgrimage and concludes that no physician is ever to decide when this pilgrimage must end (Saunders 1960b).

Conceptual Tensions and Ambiguities in Palliative Care

What becomes clear from the developments in North America and Europe as described above is that palliative care is moving back into formal health care systems. Starting off as hospice care, palliative care in the twenty-first century can no longer be identified with hospice. Rather, its organizational settings have diversified. This development has consequences, not only for the organization of palliative care but also for the meaning of the concept. We will argue below that the more palliative care is integrated with mainstream health care facilities, the more ambiguous the concept becomes.

Typically, patients enter the hospice when their prognosis is poor. But incurably ill patients on an oncology ward may have years before death and still receive palliative care. Care in nursing homes too is often provided over a period of years. In other words, the more palliative care is integrated in a variety of settings, the less it is associated with the terminal phase. As early as 1993, concerns were expressed that palliative care was no longer focused on dying: 'palliative care shifts the focus of attention away from death and there is a real danger that by talking about and focusing upon palliation, people may stop talking about and confronting the fact that the individual is going to die' (Biswas 1993 p. 135). In other words, according to the author, recent developments in palliative care posed a threat to at least one core value of hospice care, namely the acceptance of death. In light of the 2002 WHO definition that stated palliative care could go hand in hand with curative efforts, the author may have a point. In the same volume however, Ahmedzai (1993) argued that palliative care should start from the moment of diagnosis, or even earlier, when the patient is worried that he may have some serious disease. A 2000 survey among European palliative care workers showed that 60 per cent of respondents agree with the statement that palliative care begins from the time of diagnosis. A vast majority favoured full integration within the mainstream health care system (Janssens *et al.* 2002). But, if the scope of palliative care is to range from the time of diagnosis to death (or later, to bereavement care), it becomes difficult to assess what specific values are central to it.

These recent changes in the organizational forms of palliative care, its scope and the patients it serves have led to concerns. If palliative care cannot be demarcated by institution, or by the disease stage and or by pathology, then what constitutes the difference between palliative care and good medical care? Due to the integration process of palliative care into mainstream health care, will not the old ideals of hospice become blurred?

According to Bradshaw, medicine used to be a tool of hospice caregivers in alleviating pain and other symptoms. But now, due to the loss of the original spiritual values underlying hospice, medicine has become the goal of palliative care. Palliative care has become an expertize that requires knowledge and skill, but as a result, it has become unconnected to the original hospice ethic (Bradshaw 1996). Again, concerns have been expressed that the traditional hospice values are under threat due to the integration process of palliative care. Since palliative medicine has been recognized as a medical specialty in the UK, some worry that the medical domain has become dominant, and this might subvert the holistic view of hospice, aiming not only to provide medical care, but psychosocial and spiritual care in a multidisciplinary effort (Field 1994). A re-integration of hospice ideals was foreseen and hoped for. But, at least according to some, the re-integration process as it currently develops is a threat to hospice ideals.

Others hold that the integration process is the only way towards long term viability, the establishment of an adequate evidence base and access for all. Instead of the 'five star hospice care' for a selected few, palliative care for all may necessarily imply that the standard of care may be somewhat lower in the various mainstream health care settings.

One other ambiguity directly relating to traditional hospice values merits attention here. As stated above, the hospice movement has always situated itself in firm opposition to the euthanasia movement (Clark *et al.* 2002). The idea that death should not be hastened is part of traditional hospice axiology. And as late as 1994 the European Association of Palliative Care officially stated: 'We should maintain an uncompromising stand against a law that would admit the administration of death' (Roy *et al.* 1994). However, even this core value of hospice is now under debate. It is widely known that the vast majority of Belgian and Dutch physicians, whether they work in palliative care or not, are in favour of euthanasia. And the idea that legalization of euthanasia would hamper development of palliative care seems difficult to uphold as a recent report of the European Parliament rated palliative care in the Netherlands fourth best out of 27 countries. The report states: 'In general, though, the conviction that quality palliative care services are necessary if euthanasia and assisted suicide are to be legal … has been instilled in Dutch policy-makers, contributing to a well-developed legal base for these services and strong public support'.[1] This statement reflects the exact opposite of the reproaches made by opponents that euthanasia is only legal because palliative care is insufficiently developed. On the contrary, the report states, since euthanasia is legal, palliative care must be well developed. It reflects an open attitude, even if one would object to euthanasia. But irrespective of one's opinion on euthanasia, the traditional hospice value that life may not be shortened, although still part of the latest definition of palliative care, is no longer self-evident.

Critical Value Analysis and the Role of Hermeneutic Ethics

As shown above the specificity of palliative care is, at least partly, a *moral* specificity. The discomfort of the hospice movement was a moral discomfort and caregivers report that palliative care entails specific values, different from the mainstream health care system (Janssens *et al.* 2002). If that is so, moral philosophy can be helpful in further explaining the moral values underpinning palliative care. Although essentialist definitions of palliative care have become impossible, an explanation of the values and norms underpinning palliative care can contribute to demarcating palliative care from other medical practices. The demarcation of palliative care is then a moral enterprise.

We have already pointed out that the 2000 survey among palliative care workers showed a large support for the integration of palliative care into the mainstream health care system (Janssens *et al.* 2002). At the same time, as we pointed out, fears are expressed that, as a consequence, palliative care is secularizing, medicalizing and shunning death. Therefore, the question as to what the values in palliative care exactly amount to is an urgent one. As was discussed above, palliative care can no longer be associated with cancer care, terminal care or hospice care. Palliative care will in the future be given shape in a variety of medical practices, and attention will shift away from cancer patients to many more kinds of patient. In order to meet the demands of formal health care, research in palliative care will remain focused on the establishment of an evidence base. Care provided will have to take increasing account of demands posed by health insurance companies.

Furthermore, the 'emotional planning' of the modern hospices is being abandoned. Instead of relying on the co-incidental presence of pioneers and volunteers in a certain region, new palliative care units will have to take account of the demand in the region. Scientific, economic and political demands that impinge on any medical specialty will also impinge on palliative care and if palliative care is to develop further it will undoubtedly have to accommodate these demands. Already before the foundation of St Christopher's, Cicely Saunders anticipated this process. At the same time, it should be realized that the discomfort of the hospice movement with regard to care for the dying in the mainstream settings was a moral discomfort. Hospice had to turn away from mainstream health care in order to allow different attitudes and knowledge to move back in. Hospices needed time to address this distinct purpose and philosophy in order to clarify their aims and refine their practice (James 1994). Since concerns are now expressed that this distinctness of hospice or palliative care is under threat, it becomes clearer and clearer that the process of maturation also involves dangers. If it is true that palliative care is medicalizing, then palliative care runs the risk of losing exactly what is at the heart of palliative care, namely the quality of life of patients and loved ones, not only from a physical, but also from a mental, social and spiritual view. The concept of palliative care has become ambiguous and amenable to numerous interpretations.

In this respect, it is noteworthy that ethics in palliative care journals is given significant interest. At the same time, the focus is not on ethical theory but on concrete dilemmas physicians encounter in practice (Hermsen *et al.* 2001). Historical, philosophical and theological theory is largely absent. Such theory is vital if critical value analysis is to be carried out. The meaning of moral notions used may, in the context of palliative care, amount to something different than in the context of curative practices. Autonomy, for instance, may acquire specific meanings in the palliative care setting: the focus may be less on decision-making and more on enabling the patient to remain in control over his/her situation. The key aim of hospice care has always been to let the patients live until they die. What is reflected in this fundamental underpinning of hospice care has less to do with the familiar liberal view of autonomy: rather than focusing on non-interference, the goal of care as expressed by caregivers reflects a positive and dynamic notion of autonomy. Autonomy in palliative care directly relates to the patient's ability to actively give shape to his/her life and uphold a sense of control in a situation of radical dependency on others. While liberalism sees a contradiction between autonomy and dependency, hospice care sees autonomy and dependency going hand in hand (Agich 2003). Autonomy is fostered and supported through good care. Rather than a right of the patient, it becomes a goal of care and a challenge for caregivers. According to some authors, the notion of authenticity, explored extensively within existentialist philosophy, may serve as a good alternative for the notion of autonomy (Janssens *et al.* 1999). Mere provision of information is then insufficient. Rather, in deliberation with caregivers, the patient is stimulated to make choices that fit best to his/her personality, i.e. choices that are authentic.

In the palliative care literature, such critical analysis is often lacking and what makes palliative care distinct often remains unarticulated. What is lacking, in other words, is a hermeneutic perspective, combining ethical theory with everyday practice (Widdershoven *et al.* 2007). In hermeneutic ethics, practice and theory are interwoven. Theoretical notions, central in diverse philosophical or theological traditions, are interpreted in the context of concrete practical settings. The notion of restraint, for instance, was used to describe the virtuous physician in the Hippocratic tradition. It may be well equipped to further explore the attitudes of many palliative caregivers and serve as an answer to what is seen as the medicalization of palliative care. Medicine, after all, is only one realm of care (Janssens *et al.* 1999). An attitude of restraint reflects furthermore that caregivers acknowledge the boundaries of medicine. As life prolongation becomes undesirable or unfeasible, medical care overlaps with psychosocial and existential care since all forms of care have the same aim: to let the patients live. Medical decision-making in palliative care is part of a multidimensional process, and psychological and spiritual dimensions may often overrule the medical dimension.

Articulating values in palliative care requires philosophical or theological knowledge and skill but at the same time it requires experience in practice. It is however the former that is missing in the ethical literature on palliative care. And thus, the meaning of moral notions often remains unclear and new richer perspectives on palliative care are unlikely to develop.

Upon hermeneutic analysis it may appear that the meaning of a moral notion reflects a particular understanding or perspective. Other perspectives may be re-introduced in order to shed a new enriching light on the notions used. A hermeneutic understanding requires that one be willing to change perspectives and gain a broader understanding. Hermeneutics brings the particularity of current discourses to the surface, and reminds us that other discourses are possible. But again, the relevance of hermeneutics requires the connection of theory and practice, for it is only in a specific practice that notions contain particular, active meaning. So perhaps autonomy may be conceived of as self-determination in acute care, while in longer-term care settings autonomy is better conceived of as a dynamic notion. Ethicists can only assess these different meanings if they are familiar with the specific care practice and have listened carefully to the caregivers working there.

The practical relevance of hermeneutic ethics for palliative care practice is concerned with the potential to confront current perspectives with other, perhaps forgotten, perspectives. For instance, historical research in the pre-modern hospices may be instructive for palliative care today. The strong focus on spirituality in the older hospices may be confronted with the current focus on medicine. Thus, new, broader perspectives emerge that can articulate the moral experience of caregivers in practice. What's more, if theoretical notions are analyzed in their practical context, this provides the basis for an ethical articulation of what palliative care is and where distinctions with other health care practices are situated.

Hermeneutics may also be relevant for the normative debates on ethical dilemmas in palliative care. What is required for hermeneutic understanding is openness and the willingness to amend or change perspectives when there are good reasons to do so. Although hermeneutic understanding is based on dialogue (Widdershoven *et al.* 2009),this does not mean that one has to agree with everything the other is saying, nor that one has to abandon one's own presuppositions or opinions. In this sense Gadamer distinguishes hermeneutic understanding from law-like understanding (Gadamer 1960). In the latter form one categorizes the expression of the other under a general law; one is not open to what the other has to say. Yet, genuine openness to the opinion of the other is all that is required for hermeneutic dialogue. Looking back on the international euthanasia debate one has to conclude that both proponents as well as opponents understood one another in a law-like fashion.

The 1994 statement of the EAPC that was mentioned above is illustrative in this respect. The hospice movement has always constructed a sharp opposition between euthanasia and palliative care. This opposition presupposes a central role for intention, as elaborated in discussions about the doctrine of double effect. While the doctor, according to Cicely Saunders, may not *intend* to end the patient's life, (s)he is obligated to withhold or withdraw futile life prolonging medical treatments (Saunders 1995). While Saunders is in fact expressing a personal belief here, it seems as if the hospice movement considers the opposition to euthanasia an intrinsic criterion of palliative care (Gracia 2002). This idea is also evident in the WHO's definition of palliative care. An open dialogue, with respect for what other caregivers have to say, is hampered if palliative care is defined mainly in opposition to euthanasia. And proponents of palliative care have also been guilty of closed-mindedness: after criticizing euthanasia in a Dutch newspaper, one writer was accused of having 'hit thousands of caregivers right in the face' (Van Dam 1997 p. 8). Both sides seem to lack sufficient openness for hermeneutic dialogue.

More recently the polarization in the euthanasia debate seems to be decreasing. The European Parliament report is an example of increasing openness to a diversity of opinion. At least it acknowledges that good palliative care is possible even when euthanasia is accepted as a last resort. A critical, open dialogue on moral aspects of euthanasia as well as on the traditional axiology of hospice seems urgent for the further development of palliative care. Different opinions are allowed to co-exist in this debate. As long as one is willing to accept that what the other says may be relevant.

Conclusion

The integration process of palliative care in the mainstream health care system has resulted in an ambiguous and ambivalent concept. Demarcating palliative care from good medical care has become complex. Scope, patient category and setting are unhelpful since palliative care is no longer terminal, hospice, cancer care. But since palliative care originated from a moral discomfort with the way mainstream health care dealt with the dying, then the assessment of palliative care becomes to a considerable extent a moral enterprise. Moral motivations underpin the concept. And since, at least according to some, this specific morality of palliative care is now under threat, this enterprise is an urgent one. In this contribution, we have mentioned several notions and values which might be useful in this respect, such as autonomy as the actual ability to shape one's life in a context of dependency. A further step in examining the usefulness of such concepts would entail intense, multidisciplinary dialogue with those caregivers who affiliate themselves with palliative care, as well as philosophical analysis of its outcome. The historical review we have described in section 1 may also provide input for this dialogue. The process of integration, which is at the same time a process of diversification (as described in section 2), may reveal issues that need to be tackled if the essence of palliative care is to be upheld. Medicalization, addressed in section 3, may be such an issue, related to the possible shift of attention away from death. In section 4 we provided preliminary tools for value analysis: openness, dialogue and willingness to change perspectives are key words. At the same time, historical, philosophical and theological expertise is required so that different meanings of moral notions can come to the surface and facilitate the change of perspective.

We began with the observation that palliative care is a relatively young phenomenon in medicine. It is also a phenomenon that is here to stay. Fostering a dialogue about underlying values, combining theoretical knowledge and practical experience, may help to further develop the normative foundation of palliative care and contribute to its positioning in the field of healthcare.

Chapter 6

Mental Illness and Medical Ethics: Insights from Heidegger and Values-Based Medicine

Steve Ramplin and Julian C. Hughes

Introduction

Individuals who experience or care for those who suffer from mental health problems have direct personal awareness of the ethical complexity of psychiatry from a participatory perspective. Inevitably, such understanding is principally pragmatic; standard ethical theories (Deontology, Consequentialism or 'Principlism') seem lacking in relevance when faced with loss of liberty, coercive treatment or a pejoratively perceived diagnosis, to highlight some typical service-user concerns. Experience reveals important aspects of the distinctive character of psychiatric ethics. Hence, this chapter will open with a brief review of service-user perspectives. Afterwards, in an attempt to understand how the ethics of mental illness differ from those of other areas of medicine, two points will be considered. First, echoing the intimate connection between psychiatric ethics and deeper philosophical issues, this chapter will use the theories of Heidegger to bring alive the ethical dilemmas of an illustrative patient–psychiatrist encounter. Secondly, building on the case study and service-user perspectives, it will emphasize the role of values in clinical decision-making in mental health, particularly the prominent role of values that are clearly diverse. This will be explored using the principles of Values Based Medicine (VBM) (Fulford 2004). But, to reiterate, an overriding concern in this chapter is to understand in what way, or the extent to which, mental illness changes the conversation in medical ethics.

Service-User Perspectives

There is something shocking about mental illness. Many valuable first-hand accounts illustrate the experiences of mental health service-users (for example, Farmer 1983 and O'Donoghue 2009). If one considers that psychiatric ethical dilemmas are frequently related to conflicts in values emerging from interactions between individuals, typically but not exclusively those between providers and recipients of healthcare, some analysis of these kinds of narrative may assist those working in multidisciplinary mental health teams to practice more ethically, through the provision of greater understanding of patients' perspectives.

What themes do mental health service-users bring to this process? Alteration of one's sense of self is a key part of their experience. Ratcliffe (2009), in an article highlighting the indispensability of phenomenology to the understanding of existential changes in psychiatric illness, derives from several first-person vignettes, a sense of the core experience in depression. He argues that it is an alteration of one's sense of self or being in the world characterized by a painful curtailment of the possibility of connecting with anything or anyone in the world now or in the future, the temporariness of which is unappreciated at the time. This loss is aggravated by an unrelenting awareness of the possibilities presumably still enjoyed by everyone else, including (one imagines) those encountered when accessing mental healthcare.

Others have in addition emphasized a sense of struggle. For example, in a philosophical case conference built around four anonymous patient perspectives, Phillips (2004) analyzed the impact of psychopathology on narrative identity, which is a concept grounded in lived experience that owes a debt to Heidegger's insight about the importance of temporality. Thus, 'one always views one's life from a present that is forever in process and that brings at each further step a reinterpretation of the past and future' (*ibid.* p. 323). Perhaps unsurprisingly this account calls attention to the prominence in service-user stories of affect-laden descriptions of suffering, the specific quality of which was, in fact, not captured. Indeed, Phillips specifically states that any narrative notion of the self would find it a challenge 'to give adequate expression to emotion and suffering' (*ibid.* p. 323). Similarly, an interpretive phenomenological study (Johnson 1998) applied a framework of Heideggerian hermeneutic phenomenology to the analysis of interviews with previously restrained psychiatric inpatients. This study identified 'struggling' as one of two major themes, with the explicit struggle against restraint reflecting the implicit sense of struggle associated with being a person with a serious mental illness. Hence, the sense of struggle comes from the ways in which symptoms of mental illness restrict and limit one's possibilities. The second theme was 'why me?' with individuals questioning why they had been thrown into these particular limiting circumstances. Again, such perspectives are likely to be heightened when contrasted, even pre-reflectively, with the imagined circumstances of care-providers.

Davidson *et al.* (2010) examined user-led narrative interviews with 80 outpatients attending for treatment of serious mental illness. While many participants actively struggled with their illness, several additional themes emerged. Interviewees described multiple and profound losses in both social and personal dimensions that contributed to their feelings of isolation. They experienced a sense of 'just-existing', as in surviving on a day-to-day basis rather than living a life. This situation was made more poignant by the ability of many to imagine or aspire to better times ahead, and by some choosing to blame themselves, rather than any material or illness factor, as the main barrier to recovery. Many service-users perceived themselves as 'being stuck', meaning that their lives were on hold, with them neither able to return to who they used to be nor progress to who they would like to become. Participants often emphasized the importance of others in helping to steer their recovery. Many advocated a significant role to a friend, relative, volunteer, peer or professional who could guide them along the journey back to normality. Those who had found mental health services helpful described how engaged care providers had assisted them to escape mental illness and reconnect with their former lives. In contrast, those with less positive experiences told of an unsupportively narrow illness focus, with priority given to factors they saw as less central, such as symptom reduction.

Pieranunzi (1997) has examined the role mental health nurses play in service-user recovery, focusing on the lived experience of power. A key theme was power derived from the connectedness in relationships. He argued that expert psychiatric nurses unknowingly related power to an ability to understand and respond to patients intuitively on a personal level. For these nurses, 'connecting' was crucial because it invested power into 'knowing', which was considered 'powerful because when a patient (or any person) is truly known, they can respond to being known by relating in ways that enrich their life' (*ibid*: 159). Another facet of power derived from connectedness was mutuality, the notion that relationships are not unilateral but are capable of enriching the lived experience of both parties (in this case, the service-users and expert psychiatric nurses).

Typical of the intimate connection between psychiatry and philosophy, to which we will return when we consider the method of VBM, many of the themes emerging from the aforementioned service-user and professional narratives can be reinterpreted using the thinking of Heidegger. He emphasized the centrality of Being, using the German word *Dasein* to describe the simultaneity of a human being immersed in a world of things as well as possible engagements with that world. Being-in-the-World is a common thread uniting the above accounts. Each *Dasein* is thrown into his or her existence and will encounter a unique set of possibilities and limitations. For those who experience mental illness this brings certain challenges, with which mental health providers can either help or hinder. It is to a Heideggerian analysis of ethical problems arising within a framework of mental illness that we now turn.

It is worth emphasizing, however, why it is that this turn to Continental Philosophy seems appropriate. Of course, we could discuss the themes that emerge from the experience of mental illness – its effects on the sense of self, problems and possibilities associated with the presence or absence of our human connectedness, the sense of struggle, the question 'Why me?', the losses, isolation and feelings of just existing or being stuck – in terms of deontological, consequentialist or principlist approaches to medical ethics. But, first, the links between these theoretical approaches and the lived experience of mental illness are tenuous: they would have to be argued for; the theories do not really speak of the experience. Secondly, these theoretical approaches are just too theoretical. They approach the lived experience from a theoretical stance, from the stance of the disengaged observer. The Continental approach, contrariwise, both encompasses these lived phenomena as central to the problems with which it concerns itself and, moreover, does this by recognizing that our stance to these issues cannot be disengaged. To understand the issues requires that we are engaged and even shocked by them.

It is with this in mind that we present the following illustrative case, which is fictitious but based on a real (anonymized) case, of an ethically complex encounter between a psychiatrist and a service-user.

Case Study: John's Story

John, a lecturer, was referred urgently to a psychiatrist by his general practitioner following concerns raised by his daughter. On the back of a divorce from his wife of two decades, he had a four month history of gradually worsening low mood with associated lethargy, sleeplessness, poor appetite, impaired concentration and anhedonia (i.e. a loss of pleasure), such that he had long ago ceased to enjoy his job or former hobbies. Indeed, he had stopped attending work several weeks earlier, becoming increasingly isolated. The psychiatrist assessed John at home and found him sitting in the darkest corner of a room, with the curtains drawn. It was clear John was neither attending to his personal nor environmental hygiene; he was gaunt, unshaven and surrounded by uneaten takeaways. John said little during the consultation. He complained of exhaustion and an 'ache' deep within. Although he acknowledged his evident misery, he expressed no desire to change his situation. In fact, he appeared to draw a perverse pleasure from what he saw as a self-imposed confinement that he believed would continue until his death. Indeed, he said he deserved to suffer eternally, believing he deserved punishment for perceived failures in both his marriage and career. John also alluded to ideas of guilt and described feeling 'detached' from his daughter and other people in general. More alarmingly, he briefly alluded to a certain imminent end to his suffering, although when the psychiatrist asked for clarification, he refused to explain what he had meant in more detail. Toward the end of the interview, John rather brusquely dismissed the psychiatrist, accusing him of being unable to 'comprehend' his situation.

The psychiatrist diagnosed John with a severe depressive episode with somatic syndrome (implying there were also biological symptoms). John refused admission to psychiatric hospital. However, the psychiatrist was sufficiently concerned about the risk of both suicide and self-neglect that he recommended John be compulsorily admitted for several weeks to an inpatient psychiatric unit for treatment. Although John did eventually recover, he never accepted it had been necessary to deprive him of his liberty.

John's presentation and management are not atypical. Viewed through the lens of traditional biomedical ethics, provided he is competent, the decision to detain him can be understood as the elevation of beneficence over autonomy, justified by the psychiatrist's judgement that to do otherwise would incur an excessive risk of harm (suicide or death through self-neglect). This exposes him to the criticism of paternalism, with its associated neglect of the service-user's values.

Insights from Heidegger

Martin Heidegger is an influential, if still controversial, German philosopher whose thinking contributed to such diverse fields as phenomenology, existentialism and hermeneutics. In 1927, he published what is considered by many to be his greatest work, Being and Time (*Sein und Zeit*) (Heidegger 1962), a complex explication of Being, the content of which we shall shortly discuss in more detail. The on-going controversy relates to his subsequent involvement in the Nazi movement, although he later expressed covert criticism of Nazi ideology and was for some time under the surveillance of the Gestapo. During the 1930s he also underwent a conceptual shift, when he turned to the exegesis of philosophical texts and then to an examination of pre-Socratic thinking.

Using Heidegger's thought to gain a deeper understanding of the ethics of mental illness may in some respects appear odd; not only is there his onetime endorsement of Nazism, but there is also his rejection of the notion of an objective morality. Heidegger, although admitting the necessity of ethics, favoured the idea of Resoluteness, whereby *Dasein* embraces living, in which authentic decisions, meaning those where an individual strives to make his life his own, are made from extant possibilities. This is contrasted with an inauthentic existence in which one simply moves along lost in the crowd. However, this position invites the criticism of opening the door to moral anarchy. (Moral relativism, however, is a potential problem for a number of approaches in ethical theory, including VBM, which we discuss below, where a clash of values might not be settled unless appeal can be made to something beyond the values themselves.) There have been a variety of responses (for example, Hodge 1995; Lewis 2005; and Miyasaki 2007), which are united by the extent to which they attempt to provide a foundation for ethics in some aspect of Heidegger's concept of Being. Another approach has been to re-evaluate the idea of authenticity, which Taylor (1991) has argued, presupposes external 'horizons of significance' that are both shared within a community and partly constitutive of that community. Such horizons are capable of providing the objective backdrop against which resolute decisions can be evaluated as ethically better or worse. The relevant message is that Heidegger's work is not necessarily incompatible with ethics.

In addition, there is strong evidence that Heidegger believed his philosophy was highly relevant to the practice of psychiatry. In 1947, he was approached by the Swiss psychiatrist Medard Boss, initiating a lifelong friendship with regular correspondence and meetings, in which 'Heidegger strove to transcend the bounds of philosophy while Boss and his colleagues ... sought to better understand their patients and their world' (Heidegger 1987: back cover).

Before considering how his philosophy might help us to understand the ethical complexities of the clinical encounter between John and the psychiatrist, it is helpful to outline aspects of Heidegger's at times abstruse thought in more detail. As mentioned above, for Heidegger the centrality of Being is paramount – indeed, *Being and Time* (Heidegger 1962) is an attempt to elucidate the concept. He argues that *Dasein* is a being that understands it exists. *Dasein* does not exist in a vacuum, but is inextricably intertwined with all other entities it encounters in the world, as it is solely by virtue of the relationship between *Dasein* and entities in the world that anything external to *Dasein* is invested with any meaning. *Dasein* and the world are thus complementary; one cannot have meaning without the other.

Dasein is effectively catapulted (Heidegger uses the term 'thrown') into a world that is already imbued with discoverable meanings. Unlike inanimate entities, for *Dasein* Being-in-the-world offers possibilities and demands choices. Within limits, such as the restrictions imposed by external and internal confines like circumstances or genetically determined ceilings, *Dasein* is free to choose – it is whatever it decides or has decided to be.

However, we do not always deliberately decide. Sometimes, we simply go along with the flow, not really giving much active thought to what we do or why we do it. At times, we also might choose to do something we would otherwise prefer not to do in order to conform to what we believe is the expectation of the majority. To Heidegger, these positions are *inauthentic*, if necessarily prevailing as part of average everydayness. By contrast, *authentic Dasein* is being true to one's own self, making individualized choices, based on known preferences, values and ideals, instead of ceding decisions to an amorphous 'they'.

Heidegger argues that a fundamental component of *Dasein* is its state of Being-with (which relates to all other entities, including inanimate objects and other *Dasein*). A special case of Being-with is Being-with-toward-others, because some entities encountered by *Dasein* in the world are themselves *Dasein*, and therefore share the ability to understand pre-reflectively that they (and others) exist. This is so even when *Dasein* is alone because the concept of aloneness incorporates the conspicuous absence of others. Even when alone, therefore, the existent human cannot be disengaged: engagement is inherently part of *Dasein*'s Being. A criticism of Heidegger's promotion of authenticity is that it risks endorsing a type of morally unanchored self-interest at the expense of others. One response is to invoke the concept of Care (*Sorge*), which describes *Dasein*'s fundamental attitude of engagement with the world – to be in the world is to demonstrate Care. Solicitude (*Fürsorge*) is Care associated with Being-with-toward-others. A potential aspect of Solicitude is the empathic recognition that another is in need of help which one is able to provide. However, Solicitude does not imply a particular attitude and is also compatible with a self-centred approach to engaging with others. Another response to the charge that what is being set up is an ethically vacuous authentic individualism can be found in Taylor (1991):

> modes that opt for self-fulfilment without regard (a) to the demands of our ties with others or (b) to demands of any kind emanating from something more or other than human desires or aspirations are self-defeating, ... they destroy the conditions for realizing authenticity itself (Taylor 1991 p. 35).

Another final but crucial aspect of Heidegger's philosophy (prefigured in the title of his great work) needs mention. Time invests Being with meaning. *Dasein* is temporal; it has concurrent awareness of the past, the present and also of the future, meaning the multitude of emergent possibilities and the one certainty of life, namely death. For example, at any point in his depression John will have simultaneous awareness of his bleak present, of future possibilities, although it is likely his prevailing mood will limit what he imagines is attainable, and his past, though again his prevailing mood makes it probable he will selectively recall the parts of his life he looks back on with most distaste. Heidegger argues that *Dasein's* prescient awareness of death (which need not be imminent) motivates engagement with the world and roots authenticity. By contrast, the inauthentic, while aware of death, do not consider it. It becomes distant, allowing them to drift with the crowd.

John's Perspective

Can these ideas illuminate the ethical quandary evident in the interaction between John and his psychiatrist? Let us first consider the situation from John's standpoint. He appears melancholic and tormented. In common with the earlier service-user perspectives, one imagines he is plainly suffering. As *Dasein,* his sense of self seems shrunken. Certainly, his engagement with life has diminished (he is absent from work and isolative) and his state of Being-in-the-World has therefore contracted, with fewer possibilities either evident or embraced. From his darkened hideaway, it is as if he lacks Care, the desire to connect to the world which is a fundamental aspect of *Dasein.* Without Care, his Being is truncated; in John's case, he lacks concern for even the most basic entities in the world, as evidenced by his uneaten food and self-neglect. This 'loss of rapport with things', which occurs in depression, has been noted by Heidegger (1977 p. 252) and prompts the thought that Heidegger's ideas could assist a therapist to help John re-establish his Being.

In the first place, one might ask if John is acting authentically. On the one hand, his absent 'desire to change his situation' might be seen as inauthentic; he is going along with the circumstances forced by his depression. On the other hand, he also sees his confinement as 'self-imposed', suggesting a resolute decision at some level. Similarly, there is an implicit suicidal threat, surely (given the centrality of Death in Heidegger's thought) the epitome of authenticity?

> If I take death into my life, acknowledge it, and face it squarely, I will free myself from the anxiety of death and the pettiness of life – and only then will I be free to become myself. (Heidegger 1977, opening page)

However, while it could be argued that suicide may sometimes be a consequence of an authentic decision, in the context of lack of Care (i.e. where there is a disinclination to make the intrinsically human connection with the world) on account of severe depression, its authenticity is questionable. And if John's Care is deficient, any suicidal act becomes inauthentic. Of course, this knowledge is hardly likely to dissuade him (he would in all probability disagree). The important point is that this inauthenticity underlies the psychiatrist's duty to intervene. This remains the case even where there is no direct intent to end life; one can easily imagine John is also at risk of death from dehydration or starvation as a result of disengagement from Being-in-the-world. Echoing the earlier service-user commentaries, he is 'stuck'; John is so disconnected from the world, including others within it, that he cannot authentically find his way back without assistance.

Dasein alone is incomplete. Yet John's Solicitude (his attitude of Care in Being-with-toward-others) is similarly blunted. Therein lies a conundrum: how can a man as disconnected from others as John seems to be from his wife, work colleagues and students, if not entirely from his daughter or psychiatrist, reconnect sufficiently to be able to engage once more with Being?

The Psychiatrist's Perspective

Let us now consider this situation from the psychiatrist's perspective. Although the case reveals little about him, we can reasonably infer he is of similar intelligence to John. One imagines they could connect under other circumstances. When Being-with-toward-others, *Dasein* is pre-reflectively aware of its reciprocal obligations. Thus, while authentic *Dasein* can choose how and with whom to interact, the situation of Being-with-toward-others engenders certain constraints. For example, any imagined prior encounter between the psychiatrist and John as individuals would likely have adhered to well known socio-cultural rules. Similar conventions play out when doctors interact with patients (Szasz and Hollender 1956). Typically, psychiatrists work on a model of Mutual Participation. However, in John's case the interaction is closer to an Activity–Passivity model more usually associated with the non-conscious patient. To be plain: the doctor (in this case, the psychiatrist) administers to an inert patient (John, whom he detains). How might this scenario be elucidated?

It is clear from the case study that the psychiatrist struggles to connect with John as another Being. In the first place, there are unpleasant physical barriers: the gloomy room, John's poor self-care and the uneaten food. The psychiatrist surmounts these obstacles by way of Solicitude, his attitude of Care to Being-with-toward-others in the world. However, his Solicitude can be variously expressed: perhaps his ability to transcend any possible discomfiture is motivated by professionalism, altruism or even curiosity, to give three examples. The mechanism of his Solicitude is empathy, which involves seeing the existential foundations of John's misery. Yet the psychiatrist's Solicitude becomes inadequate in face of John's withered attitude of Care. Essentially, the psychiatrist experiences no reciprocity of engagement on which to found a state of Being-with; it is akin to Being-with an inanimate entity rather than another Being. One consequence is the Activity–Passivity style of interaction. Another is a distortion of the psychiatrist's experience of mutuality; while this particular interaction with John undoubtedly impacts upon his own lived experience, it probably does not do so at this point in a mutually enriching manner. One would hope that over time the psychiatrist (or other mental health professional) authentically Being-with John would lead to a good outcome, in the sense that John would feel that someone had been with him throughout.

What about the possibility of Death, Heidegger's ultimate motivator? In Being-with toward John, the psychiatrist is brought face to face via the threat of suicide and gross self-neglect with a stark reminder of the death prospect. While such reminders are frequent enough within medicine, in psychiatry they typically have the added brutality of a veil of authenticity. In medicine, death is usually related to circumstance – disease or an accident, for example. This distances the observer. Where death is related to suicide, any such comfort is less obvious. Hence the psychiatrist, in enacting his duty to prevent John's suicide (a duty derived from the inauthenticity originating in John's lack of Care) when faced with death and unreflected Solicitude, is authentic. He chooses to intervene, detaining John to impose life, at the same time quelling his own anxiety of Being associated with death. His response is, however, rooted in the duty derived from an inauthentic act. By contrast, it is interesting to consider the role of a psychiatrist faced with an authentic, or rational, suicidal intent (admittedly a controversial concept). The death anxiety undoubtedly remains, and with it some discomfort, but the justification for interfering must come from elsewhere, and there is little solace to be had from the idea of legitimate value diversity.

Does this analysis dissolve the ethical dilemma? It offers some elucidation, by way of a deepened understanding. However, where is the moral grounding? That is to say, how does the psychiatrist in a situation of un-reflected Solicitude ensure his response (which in this case is clearly coercive) is right, rather than merely his own authentic reaction to an individual apparently without Care? In other words, does the failure to connect undermine the morality of his authentic decision? One methodological approach in psychiatry to ethical difficulties originating in value diversity is the explicit consideration of the values held by others with the aim of reaching a consensus, a technique called VBM.

Values-Based Medicine

VBM is the 'theory and practice of effective healthcare decision-making for situations in which legitimately different (and hence potentially conflicting) value perspectives are in play' (Fulford 2004 p. 205). It was developed primarily from philosophical value theory as a reaction to escalating value complexity in healthcare, which is particularly evident in mental health. Fulford (1989) previously used philosophical value theory to develop the traditional fact-centred medical model into a more balanced framework incorporating both values and facts, arguing that this dichotomy, while more obvious in a conceptually complex discipline like psychiatry, is in fact present throughout medicine. Where values are shared, clinical decisions are not usually contentious; most people think pain is bad and seek both analgesia and a cure. In contrast, where values differ, decision making is more difficult. For example, in John's case it is imaginable that he might believe he will emerge stronger from his grief if he faces and overcomes it alone at home. VBM is a practical response to this complexity, much in the same way that Evidence Based Medicine was a response to the growing complexity of facts in healthcare. The ten principles of VBM are intended to assist practitioners to become more aware of the values at play in conflictual situations, since once made explicit they can be addressed. In this way, VBM is more effective than traditional biomedical ethics, which is inadequate for problems rooted in value diversity because it promulgates 'moral facts' (Fulford 2004 p. 207). The following analysis considers the effectiveness of VBM in John's case.

The first principle of VBM emphasizes the role that facts and values play in all healthcare decisions, whether concerned with diagnosis or treatment. For example, that anhedonia is a core symptom of depression has some epidemiological basis. However, deciding whether a particular patient's experience constitutes the symptom of anhedonia (and even whether anhedonia is in fact a *bad* thing, as opposed to a route to enlightenment, for instance) is the result of a complex interaction between the person describing the experience, his or her assessor and a shared cultural motif. In John's case, in addition to evident factual considerations, the psychiatrist made two implicit value judgements: first, that both the severity and range of John's complaints (including anhedonia) and the extent of his dysfunction were bad enough to warrant the diagnosis of a severe depressive episode; and, secondly, that the most appropriate intervention was enforced hospitalization, a covertly value-based judgement grounded in risk of harm. While this seems sensible enough from the viewpoint of the psychiatrist (and perhaps others), John may take a different view.

This brings the second principle into play, namely that we notice values when they conflict. John's case illustrates this nicely. One interpretation of the psychiatrist's analysis is that, notwithstanding the likely psychosocial precipitant (divorce), he has concluded that John needs urgent medical treatment for a severe depressive illness with a significant biological component. On the other hand, John's divorce and potentially linked ideas of guilt might justify his own belief that his suffering is deserved as part of a cathartic process. In other words, his value perspective could be legitimately different. On this reading, his reluctance to acquiesce to therapeutic labelling or intervention appears more understandable, while simultaneously making the psychiatrist's approach seem more heavy-handed, however well intentioned.

The third principle is that scientific progress underlies value diversity. The impetus to commit John to hospital is underwritten by a belief in the value of interventions that have arisen from the medicalization of mental disorder. The point is that without scientific endeavour there would be no treatments like antidepressant medication or electroconvulsive therapy about which to argue.

The fourth principle promotes service-user-centred practice. This does not equate to 'patientocracy'. Rather, it means that 'our first call is the perspective of the particular patient (or group of patients) concerned in a given decision' (Fulford 2004 p. 215). This principle flows from value diversity. However, even if values expressed by a particular service-user or user group differ from those held by healthcare providers (and vice versa) their respective value positions are legitimately different, at least in the sense that they are perfectly entitled to take a contradictory position. As John's case illustrates, a service-user's perspective can reasonably diverge from that of his psychiatrist. To emphasize the point: even from his position of Being-in-the-World without Care, John might conceivably feel it necessary to live through the grief of his divorce in order to become more resilient, in which case compulsory medical treatment might, in his eyes, be a retrograde step.

How to resolve such differences? The crux of VBM is the fifth so called 'multi-perspective' principle: whereas empirical methods can guide disagreements about facts to consensus, Fulford (*ibid.* p. 216) argues that divergent values can only be resolved by 'dissensus', that is 'processes that support effective action through a balance of legitimately different value perspectives'. In John's case, it does appear as if this could lead to a broader understanding. Ultimately, however, a decision is required. The psychiatrist may legitimately feel that, despite an intuitively sensible psychological explanation, John's situation remains untenable because of a suicide risk. Conversely, John may never accept the idea of compulsory hospital admission. In England and Wales, the Mental Health Act solves this dilemma democratically. While a doctor must recommend an individual's detention, a concurring non-medical professional with expertize in mental disorder is needed to activate the process, introducing a kind of values-democracy. Yet in John's case there is still a problem, originating in the disconnectedness between him and others already identified by the Heideggerian analysis. How can the process of reaching dissensus possibly proceed when the individuals involved cannot connect? Such circumstances surely require a moral arbiter, some mechanism by which to decide the proper outcome, namely what is good and what is bad?

While the remaining principles of VBM could be taken to gesture toward a solution, they admittedly do not resolve this particular problem. Principle six promotes careful attention to language in order to recognize the values influencing a problem. Principle seven advocates the use of empirical and philosophical techniques to improve knowledge of the values of others, which we otherwise tend to assume are similar to ours. Service-user perspectives are one rich source of such data, but there are many more, from reading good literature to anthropological investigation, all grist to the perspective-broadening mill. Fulford also advocates the use of philosophical methods, commenting in particular on the 'rich' resource of continental philosophy of which the Heideggerian analysis of John's case is illustrative. Principle eight advocates the use of moral reasoning to explore the 'space of values'. Engaged in this manner, applied ethical theories, like Consequentialism, Principilism and Casuistry, undergo a shift in focus that helps enlighten all the participants involved in a moral dilemma – assuming they are able to connect appropriately. Communication skills therefore have a substantive role, which is acknowledged in principle nine. Finally, principle ten shifts the onus of decision-making back from ethicists and lawyers to users and providers. However, Fulford does note that despite strident efforts, conflicts will inevitably remain as 'legitimately different value perspectives are the norm in healthcare' (*ibid.* p. 222). In this situation, he advises that the practical response may be 'leaving well enough alone'. However, as John's case illustrates, sometimes this may not be possible; if John is indeed suicidal, then leaving well alone is potentially negligent. In matters of life and death, where lies the moral compass? The commendation of continental philosophy by VBM does in fact signal a possible solution. According to Heidegger, we all ought to be engaged in Being-with-toward-others authentically in the world. This can be used to justify the same charge of moral relativism to which VBM is vulnerable. However, Taylor (1991) argues that we derive meaning from our very inter-connectedness in the public sphere.

> Things take on importance against a background of intelligibility. Let us call this a horizon. It follows that one of the things we can't do, if we are to define ourselves significantly, is to suppress or deny the horizons against which things take on significance for us ... In stressing the legitimacy of choice between certain options, we very often find ourselves depriving the options of their significance (Taylor 1991 p. 37).

In other words, our engaged Being-in-the-world reflects something vital, a horizon of significance that infuses life with meaning. Thus, even if John's decision to embrace the possibility of death was interpreted as an authentic expression of his value diversity, to do so divests it utterly of its public significance and unintelligibility. In this way, limits are placed on the liberal ideal of the right to self-determination, forestalling even the rational suicide.

Conclusions

In the introduction we wondered how the ethics of mental illness differ from those in other areas of medicine. We hope to have demonstrated that psychiatric ethics has a unique quality, intersecting on the one hand with deeper conceptual and philosophical issues, and on the other with all the complexities inherent in a discipline characterized by explicit value diversity.

Service-user perspectives figure prominently in the practice of psychiatry as compared to many other medical disciplines. However, as the theory of VBM illustrates, all healthcare decisions are arguably based on facts and values, and it is inevitable, not just in psychiatry but throughout medicine, that scientific progress will continue to open up choices that will be associated with diverse points of view. The biomedical ethicist might respond to such diversity by applying ethical theories to a problem to identify the right course of action. VBM treads a more cautious path, seeking to place patients' perspectives on an equal footing with that of professionals in order to understand the values at play and achieve an outcome that is more acceptable to all. Sometimes, it is not possible to reach such consensus. However, while VBM may lack an absolute answer, it is able to gesture toward a potential solution. Thus, while John and his psychiatrist could not agree, the application of continental philosophy brings at least some depth of understanding and consequent clarity.

Mental illness changes the conversation in medical ethics to the extent that it demonstrates our mutual connectedness as an inherent feature of our Being; thereby it shows the importance of our engagements. These include the mutual engagement of professionals and service-users, as well as our own engagement (as writers and readers of this chapter) with the dilemmas of practice. Our use of Heidegger should remind us that there is something shocking about mental illness which requires that our responses are in tune with the authenticity or otherwise of patients' positions. There is also the suggestion that our Being-with-towards-others gestures at the horizon of significance, which provides the possibility of enough objectivity to justify our decisions in despite of values diversity.

Chapter 7

Depression, Physician-Assisted Suicide and the Dutch *Chabot* Case

Christopher Cowley

In 1991, the 50-year-old Dutchwoman Mrs. Bosscher (known in the legal case[1] as Mrs. B) visited psychiatrist Dr. Boudewijn Chabot and asked him to provide the means and assistance for her to commit suicide. At that time, there was a long-standing legal convention that in the event of physician-assisted suicide (PAS) or active euthanasia (for a physically incapacitated but competent patient), the doctor would be able to defend himself against a formal charge of murder or assisting suicide by the defence of 'necessity' (in Dutch: *noodtoestand*). Such a defence still required a stringent set of substantive and procedural conditions to be met: the patient had to be suffering from a serious and identifiable somatic disease that was untreatable though not necessarily terminal; the suffering had to be 'unbearable' and 'hopeless'; the patient had to be competent enough to understand the situation and the consequences of what she was requesting, and the request had to be 'persistent'.

Mrs. Bosscher presented with a physiologically healthy body, but with deep depression. The depression was nothing new; she had been seeing psychiatrists for 20 years, but it had come to a head because of recent events. She had been married to an abusive alcoholic from the ages of 22 to 47, after which she finally left him; the elder of her two sons committed suicide when she was 45; and the younger had just died from cancer three months prior to her visit to Dr. Chabot – she was now 50. The same evening of the second son's death, Mrs. Bosscher attempted suicide by overdosing on pills that she had been hoarding for just that purpose; the attempt failed and she recovered two days later in hospital. During the three months after that, she was openly making detailed plans for further attempts, in consultation with others, including her sister, some of her friends, and her family doctor. In Dr. Chabot's opinion, Mrs. Bosscher was 'experiencing intense, long-term psychic suffering that, for her, was unbearable and without prospect of improvement' (as cited in Griffiths 1995 p. 235).

Chabot consulted seven other professionals about the matter (five doctors, a clinical psychologist and a professor of medical ethics), and took detailed notes. He repeatedly advised her to try pharmacological and psychotherapeutic treatment, but she consistently and confidently refused: all she wanted was to die. In the end he provided Mrs. Bosscher with a lethal dose of barbiturates, which she drank in the presence of him and one of her friends. He then immediately contacted the public coroner, and submitted his detailed case and discussion notes. Dr. Chabot was duly charged under Article 294 of the Dutch Penal Code, and his attempted defence of necessity was ultimately rejected by the Supreme Court three years later, in 1994. The main reason for the rejection, however, was that Dr. Chabot had failed to invite another qualified medical practitioner to examine Mrs. Bosscher for himself; importantly, the Court did not object in principle to the possibility of 'psychic suffering' henceforward being a sufficient reason to grant effective immunity to prosecution. In recognition of this fine line, the Court imposed no punishment on Dr. Chabot.

This case of 'psychiatric euthanasia' caused a certain amount of controversy, both in the Netherlands and abroad, for it seemed to be a giant leap on the oft-predicted slippery slope. In practice, during the 17 years since *Chabot*, there have never been more than three or four cases of psychiatric euthanasia per year,[2] out of an annual Dutch total of, for example, 1933 reported cases of PAS and euthanasia in the year 2005 (Buiting *et al.* 2009). Despite its rarity, the controversy continues to flare up now and then.[3]

The case is unsettling, and in this chapter I would like to explore possible reasons for its unsettling nature. This chapter is not about euthanasia *per se*; and for the sake of argument and contrast I will accept that (i) *somatic* suffering can be objectively measured, and (ii) that it can be reliably deemed sufficiently unbearable and hopeless so as to morally and legally justify physician-assisted suicide or active euthanasia. I want to argue, however, that *mental* suffering and somatic suffering are two radically distinct experiences, and that both Chabot and the Dutch Supreme Court were wrong in failing to distinguish them sufficiently: Dr. Chabot should not have helped Mrs. Bosscher to die. In reaching this conclusion, however, I want to stress two things. First, I am acutely aware of my ignorance of the particularities of the Dutch legal and healthcare systems, and indeed of the semantic nuances of the Dutch language, so my arguments should be taken as more general. Second, this is not an article about the moral permissibility or impermissibility of euthanasia in non-institutional contexts. I am primarily interested in the doctor's dilemma, while remaining agnostic on the question of whether it would be morally or rationally justifiable for Mrs. Bosscher to commit suicide on her own, or with the help of a close friend.[4]

Somatic Suffering vs. the Mental Suffering of Depression

More needs to be said about the distinction between the somatic suffering associated with a broken leg, the flu and cancer, and the mental suffering associated with depression: after all, isn't all suffering ultimately mental? The difference has to do with the link to events in the world. The link is clearest in the case of physical trauma: the fracture is caused by the tree's impact on the skier's leg. Although the suffering is ultimately mental if we assume with the scientist and philosopher some sort of identity between mind and brain, phenomenologically it is the *leg* that hurts. And it is this first-personal phenomenology that interests me here, more than a third-personal scientific account. Central to the first-person experience is precisely the distinction between self and world, that is, between me on the one hand, and the tree, the impact, the broken leg and the pain on the other. (This is not to assume an implausible dualism, with the self as essentially separate from the body; it is merely to make a point that the suffering of a broken leg is *localized*.)

A more complicated case of somatic suffering is that brought about by an invisible pathogen (such as an airborne flu virus) or by abnormal cellular growth and subsequent organ failure (cancer). In both cases, the patient first notices the suffering and the superficial symptoms, and uses the subsequent scientific picture to help make sense of the suffering; even if the patient is not a scientist, enough of the process can be understood metaphorically by imagining, say, aggressors overcoming defences. Throughout, however, the distinction between self and world remains intact: I still have my plans and projects, but their progress has become restricted, cramped, hindered by my dysfunctional body in the world. The cause of the pain remains clear enough: a foreign object, a malfunctioning component, a disease entity. I can still use the language of possession: I *have* a broken leg, the flu, cancer, and it is causing me pain. (It is true that once the somatic suffering reaches extreme levels, then the distinction between self and world starts to blur, and I can only scream. But in the Dutch euthanasia cases I am assuming that the patient is still able to repeatedly and consistently articulate their wish to die, which is one of the conditions for assistance.) Somatic medicine provides a detailed taxonomy of injury and disease, allowing inductive comparison and contrast with past and present cases, so that the objective symptoms corroborate and explain the subjective reports. Different people with the same stage two liver cancer will, other things being equal, have the same symptoms, the same prognoses, and the same treatment options available. Even if the precise nature of the somatic suffering may differ from patient to patient, the suffering is anchored in the general scientific description.

Even if there is always a certain amount of guesswork in diagnosis and prognosis, a post mortem examination can then confirm or falsify a good deal about the disease and its attempted treatment retrospectively. This point about confirmability is important, because the assumption of somatic medicine is that there is a clear set of objective facts underlying the suffering, and that any uncertainty in diagnosis and prognosis is merely epistemic, based on the limitations of science and the difficulty of intrusive testing on a living body.

The link to the world is also important for our own empathetic understandings – and moral judgements – of other people's somatic suffering resulting from their encounters with the world. Not only can I confidently understand most of what it feels like when you suffer a scraped elbow, a knee to the groin, an ear infection or a burn, but I can also sometimes confidently reproach you for your complaints: 'keep walking, you big wimp, it's just a blister'. In this sense, there is an objective aspect to unbearability: we would say that the hiker was mistaken in claiming his blistered foot to be unbearable. Guy Widdershoven agrees: 'Dutch physicians will not be satisfied with a simple declaration by the patient on the subject of their suffering. They will interpret such declarations in the context of the patient's total situation' (Widdershoven 2002 p. 99).

Even when I have no direct experience of a severe disease such as cancer, I can imaginatively extrapolate using the usual metaphors to achieve some vague idea of what you must be going through and I can admire your courage in keeping a cheerful disposition. All of this serves to anchor the suffering patient in the world: the ordinary world of dangerous trees and cars, the scientific world of causal explanations and invisible pathogens, and the moral world of praise and blame.

Things are much less clear with the mental suffering of depression. In what follows, I'm going to focus entirely on depression, since I am not sure how far my thesis would apply to other kinds of mental illness such as compulsions or delusions or dementia or multiple personality disorders, and the phenomenology of the various mental illnesses varies so much, and is often so complicated, especially in its effects on the will. And while depression is basically intelligible, since we have all had feelings of sadness or worthlessness or hopelessness, it is not clear whether other mental illnesses are so readily intelligible or imaginable. (Perhaps the most extreme forms of depression are not intelligible, but I am taking Mrs. Bosscher's depression to be sub-extreme.) I'm also going to avoid the case of bipolar depression, where a single agent's response to the same set of facts can vary markedly in time; for here it is much more plausible to speak of an underlying somatic cause.[5]

Mrs. Bosscher's depression, on the other hand, was brought about by intelligibly depress*ing* events in her life, and for this reason George Graham (1990) would call her depression 'justified' – and I'm going to follow his usage. (Other terms for the same class are 'reactive' or 'exogenous'.) Now it is tempting to consider depression to be, *by definition*, a mental illness that is sufficiently serious to render the patient legally incompetent, to render PAS requests invalid and irrational, and to reject all possibility of justification. My own response to this sceptical position comes simply from having known justifiably depressed people who were very much competent; like other sceptical claims, I'm not sure how much this one can be philosophically refuted, and I'm not going to try.

I say that Mrs. Bosscher's depression was 'brought about' rather than 'caused' by events precisely because I want to emphasize that Mrs. Bosscher is *interpreting* those events in terms of her own life. Already this marks an important distinction between mental and somatic suffering. The tree, and the skier's brute impact with that tree, requires no interpretation. Interpretation only comes in later on, when the skier has to decide what sort of a role to allow the suffering to play in his life, for example whether he will ignore it or draw others' attention to it. The case of somatic diseases such as cancer is more complicated, since the pain in my abdomen has to be medically interpreted (diagnosed); but this interpretation comprises a strictly causal story, making reference solely to the general facts of the human body-machine and to laws of nature, not to specific facts of the patient's life. Even when the diagnosis is not clear, the nature of two doctors' disagreement is very different from the sort of disagreement that Mrs. Bosscher's sister might have with her about the conclusions that she draws from her sons' deaths. For completeness, I should mention an important class of 'grey' cases, involving perceived non-medical causes of somatic disorders, as when I interpret my cancer as divine punishment for earlier transgressions. Insofar as this leads to mental suffering and not merely somatic suffering, then what I say below about depression will also apply to such cases.

The concept of justification refers to some sort of shared standards or norms. In the case of depression, the idea is that certain familiar events will justify depression in any human life: unemployment, bereavement, debt, imprisonment, etc. Insofar as a depression is justified, then it is intelligible to other people once the events are described. Not only will such events justify the depression, they also account for its phenomenology: the depressed person's consciousness is filled *not* with a disease entity, not with some 'thing' called depression, but with the event-objects themselves.[6] If I ask Mrs. Bosscher'why are you depressed?' her answer will refer to her sons and to her relationship with them; she is suffering not from depression but from their death. Whereas if I ask the cancer patient 'why are you suffering?' they will reach for a scientific causal account, or perhaps a religious causal account – or they may not understand the question.

There is of course a parallel here between the vulnerability of human lives to general types of personal disasters and the vulnerability of human bodies to certain general types of injury and disease. However, the point about the centrality of interpretation is important here, for the depressive response is radically *individuating* in a way that somatic suffering is not. Not only is there empirically a much narrower range of particular responses to a broken leg than to the death of a loved one, but the precise contours of a particular person's grief will depend greatly on that person's character and background, on their relationship to the loved one, on the capacity of their other relationships and projects to sustain them through the grief etc. Indeed, there is sometimes a degree of surprise in that the person ends up grieving much more than they or others would have predicted while the loved one was alive. We might therefore say that depressing events, much more than other kinds of adversity (including somatic illness), reveal the character of the person suffering the events, and reveal the deeper nature of her relationships with others, living and dead.

Depression and Suicide

If we can accept that Mrs. Bosscher's depression is justified, there is now a *separate* question about whether Chabot would be justified in assisting her suicide (Graham distinguishes the questions on p. 407), and I shall argue that he would not. Let us return to the criteria of the Dutch convention: the suffering has to be 'unbearable' and 'hopeless'. Hope is an attitude toward the future: if I am genuinely hopeful, then any present adversity can be borne. But for hope to be sensible and not naïve, it has to bear some relationship to objective probabilities. So once again we find a radical difference between the hopelessness of cancer and the alleged hopelessness of Mrs. Bosscher's depression. A somatic illness usually conforms to a type, which can be observed across populations and across time: this means that predictions can be made more or less reliably, based on different treatment options, and compared to the option of non-treatment. Certain treatments can be withdrawn or withheld because they have been inductively revealed as hopeless (in the sense of futile), or overly burdensome, in a sufficient number of sufficiently similar past efforts. Although the precise definition of futile could be the subject of reasonable disagreement between equally well-informed doctors, there has to be enough agreement in the profession about most treatment decisions in order to teach the relevant generalizations to the next generation of medical students.

Justified depressive responses to the same event type vary so widely because they individuate the patient so much, and therefore the particular course of the patient's depression is *essentially* unpredictable. After all, many people suffer a family member's suicide without becoming suicidal themselves. In addition, pharmacological treatments for depression are themselves so patient-specific, and seem to be evolving so rapidly, that it is tempting to say that there are always reasonable grounds for hope that a future treatment might work well enough after trial and error. Psychotherapeutic treatments take a longer time because the therapist needs to get to know the patient well, but again there is no reason in principle to think that psychotherapy will not work well enough eventually. And yet Mrs. Bosscher confidently rejected all the treatments that Dr. Chabot repeatedly offered. It is not clear what to make of this refusal. On the one hand it is of course the competent patient's right to refuse any treatment, for any reason. Presumably she thought that no amount of treatment could change the situation and bring her sons back to life; in that sense all treatment for her was futile, and just served to prolong her suffering. On the other hand she wanted assistance from the medical profession, and the profession could surely have made such assistance conditional on at least trying the treatment, especially since the treatment in question would probably not be anywhere near as burdensome as, say, chemotherapy; to refuse to even try treatment comes uncomfortably close to a sulk. Indeed, the Dutch Medical Association's Disciplinary Committee rebuked Chabot for not making a 'more vigorous attempt to persuade her to try antidepressant medication' (cited in Burgess and Hawton 1998 p. 117). And the Dutch Supreme Court claimed that Chabot 'ought to have considered treating her with antidepressants, if necessary against her expressed refusal' (Berghmans

1998 p. 133). (It is not clear what the committee meant by 'vigorous', nor what the Court meant by 'against her refusal'. Were they recommending that she be declared incompetent, incarcerated, and then forcibly treated, for example?)

Mrs. Bosscher sincerely believes her condition to be sufficiently unbearable and hopeless to justify suicide. But in the absence of corroborating somatic conditions with clear inductively-justified prognoses, I suggest that there are no grounds to consider the depression hopeless in any demonstrable sense. Although the coming weeks and months will no doubt be hard, and the view from the present is bleak, there is no reason in principle to think that she is incapable of discovering new sources of value, new relationships or activities to fill the thirty odd years that she can still expect to live in good somatic health. Such a view of the future is essential to most of the medical profession, but particularly to psychiatry. While medical optimism can be corrupted by an obsession with technological rescues long past the point of futility and dignity, it is much harder to speak of futility in treating Mrs. Bosscher's kind of depression, because somatic illness is simply and brutally caused by the insistent biological facts of the world, while Mrs. Bosscher's depression relies in part on what she makes of the facts of the world. Psychiatry's 'optimism' (if this is the best word) is grounded in the widespread belief among non-doctors that suicide *is* something to be prevented as far as possible, that the life of the somatically healthy suicidal person can never be as hopeless as she thinks, and that those friends and family who fail to prevent a suicide will be very likely to blame themselves for not foreseeing and helping enough (see Warnock and Macdonald 2008 pp. 22–23). The only reluctant exception to this widespread view of suicide, I suggest, would be a suicide designed to end a life marred by irremediable *somatic* suffering.

Burgess and Hawton (1998 p. 117) consider the semi-fictionalized example of Robin, a 20-year old student devastated and suicidal after rejection by his girlfriend. Here we have justified depression, but there is clearly no way that any Dutch doctor would agree to assist the boy's suicide, no matter how sincerely unbearable and hopeless Robin considered his own suffering; for there are good reasons to hope, even if he cannot yet see those reasons. So this is a paradigm of what any legalized PAS system has to avoid. It is perhaps unfair to compare Mrs. Bosscher to Robin, but Dr. Chabot needs a clinically (and philosophically) robust way to distinguish the two, since the basis of both requests would ultimately be the patient's feelings and beliefs. For in the same way that the doctor could tell Robin 'these feelings will pass, you will discover other women', why can Chabot not tell Mrs. Bosscher 'these feelings will pass?' Things would be different if Mrs. Bosscher had a terminal illness and simply did not have *time* to discover new sources of values, new ways to go on living; things would be different if she had a somatic condition that would continue generating unbearable pain with no prospect for imminent release. But somatically, she is still in the middle of her life, just like Robin. We could argue that Robin has his whole adult life before him, while Mrs. Bosscher has the bulk of her working life, at least, behind her; she wouldn't be able to start a new career, for example. But this seems too thin a difference on which to base a policy of life and death.[7] In the Dutch system, the patient and the doctor are supposed to work together through to the conclusion that there is 'no option' but to end the patient's life in order to prevent further suffering (Widdershoven 2002). I'm finding it difficult to see, in the case of a depressed patient, how a doctor can ever come to this conclusion.

Mrs. Bosscher might well respond that all this talk of hope is just whistling in the wind, that all these judgements about the future by well-meaning doctors and philosophers are irrelevant because nobody else finds themselves in *her* life; nobody can understand just how close she was to her sons, just how much of her life was wasted in marriage to an abusive drunk. Precisely because she is the one who has to live on outside the therapist's consultation room, to get through the long sleepless nights, to force herself out of bed in the morning, to get through the weeks and months, this means that her wishes must carry a certain authority, including the authority required to have one's persistent suicidal wishes taken seriously. If the Dutch state has already decided *not* to respond to the suicidal cancer patient with the condescending recommendation that 'others have learned to live with cancer, and so can you', then she would see no relevant difference here. Besides, it should be remembered that Mrs. Bosscher, unlike Robin, had *already been* depressed for the better part of 20 years, had tried different treatments, and had been holding on only for the sake of her sons. So it is not as if her depression had suddenly descended, perhaps implying that it could suddenly lift again if only the psychiatrist can stall her for long enough. No, if any depression can be termed hopeless it was surely Mrs. Bosscher's and this is what Dr. Chabot judged it to be. Psychiatry had already tried to help her, and had evidently failed; in rejecting Dr. Chabot's offer of further treatment, Mrs. Bosscher knew what she was talking about. In addition, can we not credit Mrs. Bosscher with a certain degree of self-knowledge after 30 years of adult life?

It will also be objected that for Chabot to refuse Mrs. Bosscher would be to abandon her at her moment of greatest need; and would be to condemn her to a suicide that would very likely be messy, violent, and probably unfairly traumatic to others (e.g. to those who find the body). It must not be forgotten that Mrs. Bosscher had already attempted suicide on the same evening of her second son's death and was already planning to make further attempts. The standard response to this still holds, however: that the medical profession cannot give in to what is effectively blackmail. 'Kill me cleanly, or I will kill myself messily' should be rejected as a threat in the same way as the junkie's plea to the pharmacist 'give me the drugs or I will steal them'. But the argument from abandonment actually cuts both ways. In the first version, the doctor is negligent for abandoning the patient when she needs help to kill herself. But in the second version, if the doctor concurs with her decision that life is indeed hopeless, this could itself be seen as abandonment – from the perspective of the family and of the medical community. It could also be seen as abandonment from the perspective of the *hesitant* patient (i.e. not Mrs. Bosscher): 'even my GP, who has always been on my side, agrees that I should die. Now I'm just wasting his time'. Part of the doctor's job is, simply stated, to reinforce the will to live and to flatly deny the will to die. This is entirely compatible, it should be stressed, with the transformation of the doctor's role from curative to palliative efforts, and with the withdrawal of treatment that is now futile or overly burdensome after a somatic illness has progressed too far. But the claim that a depression, however justified, has gone 'too far' is much more problematic and controversial, and it suggests that a Dutch doctor should err on the side of refusing suicidal requests.

Besides, in refusing to assist her suicide, it is to be assumed that the Dutch healthcare and social welfare systems would step in to ensure that she was *not* abandoned: treatment and support would be available. So just because she wants the suicide does not mean that a refusal will constitute abandonment, for it has yet to be established that she has a right to assistance with the suicide on the grounds of unbearable and hopeless suffering. In the same way, the refusal does not constitute a 'condemnation' to years of misery; at some point the state has to step back and say: 'it's your life, you have to make the best of it'. Many people are miserable, more or less justifiably, and the state cannot be expected to guarantee happiness. It may come to pass, after the state has stepped back, that Mrs. Bosscher cannot bear it any longer, but the expression of the unbearability of her suffering has to be the fact that she makes her *own* plans and efforts to commit her *own* suicide, that the suicide be something difficult to accomplish, and that she do it in defiance of the reassuring optimism of her family and her doctors.

The Conversation Between the Doctor and the Patient

It might be felt that I have not yet satisfactorily responded to the claim that Mrs. Bosscher's depression, precisely in virtue of the 20-year history of her suffering, is sufficiently hopeless to justify assistance with her suicide. In order to build on my response, I want to imagine the possible conversations between her and Dr. Chabot.

In a 2002 article, Raphael Cohen-Almagor asked a fascinating question to a number of Dutch doctors. Instead of the more familiar questions that we find in discussions of euthanasia, questions such as 'Do you agree with the legal permissibility of euthanasia?' or 'Would you perform covert euthanasia if a competent patient requested it?', he asked: 'Should doctors *suggest* euthanasia to their patients?' Such a suggestion does not need to be as blatant as the used car salesman's pushiness, of course; it could merely be a certain emphasis on a certain word, as in 'are there any *other* options you'd like to discuss?' In the Dutch context, doctors would be wary of being too pushy, but when the doctor knows that the patient knows that euthanasia is legal, the issue is already on the table, so to speak, and the question is whether the doctor can subtly draw attention to it if the patient seems to hesitate for whatever reason.

In order to understand the problem, we might consider a well-known distinction in the theory of rights: (i) under one conception a person *has* a right to an option, and is aware that he has that right, (ii) under another conception a patient *is offered*, by an appropriate authority, an option to which he has a right. It is a mistake to think there is never any meaningful difference between these. And in most areas of human activity there may not be any such difference: if I have a right to have a lawyer present when I am being interrogated by the police, for example, then the police should be obliged to offer me one, and to offer me one not as a favour but as a recognition of that right. I should never be in the situation where I have to demand the lawyer. Only in this way can the temptations of police power be appropriately curbed, and can individuals resist the inevitable intimidation of the interrogation environment.

Now strictly speaking no Dutch citizen has a legal right to euthanasia, and no Dutch doctor has a legal duty to provide it. But insofar as a Dutch citizen understands and fulfils the criteria and conditions that will generate the situation of 'necessity' required to immunize a volunteer doctor from legal prosecution, then it may be said that this citizen is in the position to make a *de facto* legitimate claim. So it is in the context of this relationship between patient and doctor that Cohen-Almagor's question has to be understood. Once again, it is important to remember that the doctor is not offering a service to a confident customer on a take-it-or-leave-it basis: the patient is at one of the most vulnerable points of her life, in Mrs. Bosscher's case confused and disoriented about many of her deeper values – and she is quite literally desperate. But Cohen-Almagor argues, against the opinion of some of the doctors he interviews, that euthanasia should always be a last resort, and that this can only be ensured if the doctor is always on the back foot within the conversation: even if the patient fulfils all the criteria, she should still have to demand it, without prompting, and then to demand it again, and again. Only in this way can the doctor be sure that her wish is authentic.

Although Cohen-Almagor was talking about euthanasia in general and not about psychiatric euthanasia, his argument has important ramifications for the distinction I am trying to draw between the appropriate responses to somatic suffering and mental suffering. For I agree with him that psychiatric euthanasia should be prohibited, while allowing that patients can make a legitimate claim for euthanasia in response to unbearable and hopeless suffering from somatic illnesses. And I agree with Cohen-Almagor that doctors should not suggest euthanasia to patients such as Mrs. Bosscher (or even hint at it), but I disagree with him when it comes to patients with somatic illnesses within the Dutch context.

The point about somatic illnesses is that in the Netherlands the *political* debate about somatic suffering has been settled, and there is no serious movement for reform. It is discussed openly in public, and every elderly person will know about the possibility. It is the patient who has already made the first move – the authentic first move – by contacting a doctor who is a volunteer member of the Dutch Association for Voluntary Euthanasia. By the time they enter the doctor's surgery, they have already thought about it and discussed it with friends. If the patient is reticent, this is not from any shame or stigma that would have prevented her from coming to the consultation in the first place; it is more from embarrassment about discussing such a private matter with a stranger, and so the doctor's breaking the ice may indeed be appreciated. But here again my point about the separation of self and suffering comes in: the patient's somatic suffering has the same status, within her perspective, as the patient's somatic illness. They are both part of the shrinking world, and therefore localized and intertwined: to discuss the illness is to discuss the suffering. The doctor and the patient can discuss the suffering as if it were separate from the both of them, and they can reach a conclusion together on the best course of action to deal with that suffering.[8]

In contrast, consider again the encounter between Dr. Chabot and Mrs. Bosscher. In Griffiths' discussion of the case, he states: 'in letters and discussions with [Dr. Chabot], she presented reasons for her decision clearly and consistently, and showed that she understood her situation and the consequences of her decision' (Griffiths 1995 p. 235). What sort of *reasons* could these be? Obviously she would start by describing the relevant facts of her situation, especially how attached she was to her sons, and that the sons are now dead. Those facts certainly justify her depression, but are they enough to justify suicide, to persuade Dr. Chabot to assist her? The only reason that she seems able to offer for this further step is 'because I don't want to live without them'. The problem is that this is not a statement about the world, this is a statement about her. And so if Chabot agrees with her request, he is effectively making a judgement about *her life*, not about her suffering; he thereby crystallizes her interpretation of her own life without sufficient objective warrant, and entirely rejects the possibility that she might be mistaken. I consider this terribly cruel and deeply irresponsible.

To put it another way, the crucial difference between a somatic patient and Mrs. Bosscher is that the somatic patient, I suggest, at least in the vast majority of cases, *does not want to die*. If their condition could be treated, if the pain could be reduced, if some degree of functionality could be restored to their body, etc. – then they would live on. (It is true that some somatically ill people are also weary of life, or exhausted by the struggle, and so genuinely do want to die.) Mrs. Bosscher's body is fine, but she doesn't want to live on without her sons: she wants to annihilate herself. The desire to annihilate oneself is deeply mysterious. As such the somatic patient's request for euthanasia is easier to make sense of, and easier to respect.[9]

I have been arguing against a medical doctor, with all the state's recognition and the profession's moral authority, assisting the suicide of a justifiably depressed patient. However, nothing in what I have said would condemn a friend or family member helping that patient to commit suicide in a non-institutional capacity. For in such cases it would be clear that the friend could perhaps know the patient well enough to make such a serious decision, and to articulate an authoritative judgement on what is best for her. In addition, the friend, unlike the doctor, will be implicated in the suicide, for they will be losing a friend in the process and this will add moral seriousness to the decision. In principle the Dutch doctor is meant to get to know the patient before making a decision about assisting suicide, and often the doctor will have been the patient's family doctor of many years. But if the doctor knows the patient well enough to be her friend, and therefore well enough to assist her with her suicide when the patient claims to be suffering from unbearable depression, then the doctor should offer such help off-duty, as it were.

Of course the assisted suicides of depressed people would have to be investigated to make sure there was nothing close to murder, but the present legal arrangement in the UK[10] and many other countries would seem to allow an official prohibition against euthanasia to co-exist with a refusal to prosecute cases of compassionate assistance between, for example, long-married spouses.[11]

Part Three

Autonomy and Autonomous Decision-Making

Chapter 8

Autonomy: Presumptively Precluding Consequentialism in Medical Ethics

D. K. Levy

Introduction

Autonomy is among the core values in the modern, ethical practice of medicine. The challenge is finding ways to express the value of autonomy in practice, when a would-be patient presents himself to a practitioner. He does not present as a problem to be solved or improved, but as a person asking for help. Sometimes help is a response like a service; for example, you have an astigmatism, here is a prescription for glasses, get glasses. Other times, the response is a choice of assistance, for example, between surgery and drug therapy, with consent sought for assumed risks. But the most challenging aspect of the request for help is to respond with the proper form of attention to the patient, because it is through forms of attention that we express the value of autonomy.

Respect is one form of attention in which one defers to the patient's autonomy, for example, his rejection of drug-based pain management. Respect, as a form of attention, is not simply acknowledging a patient's rights under the law and tailoring treatment to fit within these. Rather, respect is expressed by withholding judgement or prejudice, by the attempt to recognize another's perspective – though not every perspective can command respect. Pity, when appropriate, is another form of attention to a person, his life, and his own conception of his life. When someone, through pride, cannot accept the scale of his infirmity, because to do so would threaten his sense of self, then responding with pity values his autonomy and is expressed by not talking down to him or giving truths that are a violence to his self-deception. Mercy is another form of attention, in which one acts contrary to what is indicated, for example, by the patient's stated desire or by clinical best practice. However, it is only mercy when it originates in attention to the particular situation – his needs, his history, for example that he is a Holocaust survivor – of the person who presented himself for help, as a patient.[1]

I assume that the ethical practice of medicine should aspire to be a home to respect, pity and mercy among other forms of attention, as desirable expressions of the value of autonomy. I shall argue that consequentialism as an ethical theory is blind to the value of autonomy. It is formally blind in its structure. It is materially blind because its conception of persons forecloses ethical responses like pity, respect or mercy. If I am right, then there is reason to be chary of consequentialist reasoning in those areas of medical ethics in which concerns of autonomy are central. Consequentialism seems a natural fit for medical ethics, but if I am right about consequentialism's blindness to autonomy then we ought presumptively to preclude it in favour of deontological approaches.[2]

I shall begin by explaining autonomy's wider importance in areas of medical ethics concerned with quality of life, in addition to its narrower importance for issues of consent. In the next section I shall suggest that consequentialism seems better suited to medical ethics than deontology. However, I offer two arguments that consequentialism cannot accommodate autonomy. I then consider several objections to these arguments the answering of which reveals how consequentialism constrains the ethical responses of medical practitioners. My argument and conclusion are limited in scope, which I try to indicate in the final section. I shall conclude that for an important domain of ethical challenges, the presumption ought to be against consequentialist reasoning.

Autonomy

Autonomy has become important in medical ethics as a reaction to the paternalism of the past in which doctors often decided what was best for patients. The value of autonomy is expressed in this context by emphasizing that would-be patients must give their informed consent to their treatment. It is well understood that medical practitioners, when they interact with another person in the practitioner/patient relationship, do so in ways that would be peculiar in most other contexts. So of course autonomy is important in seeking the consent of those people practitioners would make patients, of those who suffer medicine. Consent in this sense acknowledges that the patient has authority over his body and gives permission for his treatment.

There is another source for the importance of autonomy in medical ethics that does not arise from narrow issues of consent. Autonomy is central to someone making his life his own; to giving it the character he wishes; to giving it a coherence, structure or purpose reflective of his will. For example, someone may wish his life to be one of service to others. Someone may aim to snub authority in what he does, prizing pleasure over all else.

The life of an aesthete is another example. More generally, someone's life is his own when it is imbued with his values and aims – pleasures, interests, recognized obligations – those things he finds motivating and those things by which he motivates himself. The paternalism of the past was objectionable because it imposed value judgements into another's life.

Autonomy is central to someone's life being a good one by his own lights at least. A good life is one in which, at a minimum, the subject is not inert within his life. That is, in a good life one is motivated or motivates oneself by one's interests and values. A life is better when, among other things, one succeeds in realizing the objects of one's motivations. This conception of a good life is very thin, though it is sufficient to explain that in choosing one treatment over another, someone is exercising their autonomy in a way that is not solely consent. Rather, selecting one treatment over another is one way in which someone can make his life his own or an expression of his interests, aims or values.

There is no agreement about what makes a good life, about what, as debates sometimes put it, makes a life worth living. If there were, perhaps considerations of autonomy would be second to imperatives to make lives better. One reason for the lack of agreement is that human physiology underdetermines what makes a good life. It is questionable whether the facts of human physiology are such that an optimum in physiological growth or function could be determined by some analysis. Even if it were possible, it is plain that a human life is not identical with physiological function, that optimal physiological function is no more than a part of an optimal human life. A human life comprises also one's social life, one's successes or failures, one's sentimental life and much else.

This truth is self-evident. If it were not true, then someone in a coma, whose physiology were kept functioning optimally, would have a *better* life than someone who was not in a coma but was physiologically sub-optimal; or someone who was kept in prison with optimal physiological function would be better off than the person in society with sub-optimal physiology; or someone who was a failure in everything he attempted but blessed with optimal physiology would be better off than a successful person with sub-optimal physiological function. To claim that these comparisons favour the physiologically better off is absurd.

The situation is not improved if we take not human physiology but the idea of a human being as a being of a certain kind, where that kind has certain qualities or capacities characteristic – perhaps criterial – of being that kind. Physiological capacities would be among these, but in addition there would be social, sentimental and intellectual capacities. It is even more doubtful that from this complex of capacities there is an analysis that would identify an optimum for lives of beings of this kind, viz. the human kind. There are capacities that confound such an analysis, like imagination or style, where the very idea of an optimum capacity or the optimal exercise of the capacity is problematic.

Aristotle's *Nicomachean Ethics* is perhaps the best and most famous attempt to take seriously the idea that a human kind suggests a function or purpose by which one might attempt an analysis for an optimal life. It is arguable whether this was Aristotle's intent, but he certainly took it that humans were a natural kind with a characteristic function or purpose. Moreover, he proposed that there was an optimum in the application of each human capacity that was the median between excess and privation. For example, courage is the median between foolhardiness and cowardice. Aristotle held that if a person's human capacities were functioning at the median of each, then, absent chance, he would flourish, that is, live a good human life.

Granting that Aristotle was right in every aspect of his account, there are yet things left undetermined for a good life. If Aristotle has not accounted for everything, there must yet be scope for someone to make his life his own even if by Aristotle's lights he is flourishing. I offer two examples where Aristotle's account falls short. First, Aristotle's account seems neutral with regard to the content of a life. Courage, for instance, is good for what one may meet in life, but possession of courage is of itself not motivating, nor is it in any way indicative of what to do with one's life. Purpose must be added to an otherwise flourishing life, by for instance taking one's courage into martial endeavour or challenging dogma.[3]

Second, there are personal qualities that are not practical capacities, by which I mean that they are not essentially directed at successfully realizing one's actions. For instance, optimism/pessimism and seriousness/superficiality are not themselves capacities for action or judgement, nor are they extremes of related capacities. Yet each will give its possessor's life a distinctive character, however much that life is already flourishing. Put another way, neither optimism nor pessimism necessarily contributes to *whether* one flourishes, but the optimist and the pessimist will flourish differently.

The above argument establishes that with regard to comparisons of the quality and character of human lives, there is an ineliminable gap that cannot be filled with facts or their analyses. Therefore, no domain of knowledge, medicine or otherwise, encompasses an optimum for how a life should go. It is not therefore surprising that there is no agreement on what a good life is.

Into this gap – into this lack of agreement – must enter someone's autonomy, for it is his life and the motivations for it must be his own. The importance of autonomy is not therefore acknowledged in full by respecting someone's authority over his own body. The importance of autonomy is acknowledged by allowing that the *exercise* of autonomy is integral to a good life because a good life for an individual must originate in that individual. Exercising one's autonomy is the origin of a good life.

There are other routes to similar conclusions regarding the importance of autonomy in relation to how a life's qualities make it a good life.[4] In a modern liberal society, the liberty to conduct one's life according to one's own ideas is a founding idea, the basis for a divide between the public and private spheres. It is on this basis that political power is limited to the public sphere, leaving the private sphere to each autonomous individual. Where once religious verities were an authoritative guide to living, in our post-modern age the claim to singular authority about how to live is at least immediately subject to challenge if not wholly discredited.

Autonomy is essential to the most basic forms of interpersonal regard or disregard, in which we find the distinctive character of human life in contrast to animal life. For we praise and blame people; we hold them responsible; we admire or disdain them; we recognize their virtues, dignity or grace. These are not our relations with animals. These relations would not be possible if we thought that other people were automata or that their conduct was the product of drugs, or being in thrall to another's authority or dogma. It is essential for these forms of regard or disregard – often called respect – that someone is self-determined and not other-determined. This insight was most famously expressed by Kant, although it is a truth of common experience and a favourite literary theme.[5]

In sum, while it is common to acknowledge the importance of autonomy in medical ethics in the narrow sense of consent, my intention has been to amplify that importance as well as widen the scope and foundation of its importance. If I am right, then it shows that autonomy in this wide sense is of significant importance in any application of ethics in domains concerning quality of life, that is, the qualities contributing to a good life.

That is a coarse specification. These domains must be further refined as encompassing quality of life where the *exercise* of an individual's autonomy is the origin of the conception of and pursuit of his quality of life. In short, autonomy is to the fore when decisions must be made based on a conception of a good life. We succeed in recognizing the importance of autonomy when we succeed in ensuring that the conceptions of a good life considered are autonomous expressions of the person about whom decisions are to be made.

Consequentialism

I have shown the importance of autonomy. My overall purpose is to show that consequentialism is blind to autonomy. Before giving arguments to that effect, it is important to establish why consequentialist reasoning so often features in applications of ethics, particularly medical ethics.

It is natural to think that applied ethics – applications of ethics – are practical in nature, because it is to practical problems that the ethics are *applied*. By practical problems I mean problems in which there is a desired outcome, but the means to the achievement of that outcome is somehow problematic. It is a practical problem how to cross a raging river when possible solutions may not work or are too risky. Practical domains are defined by the techniques whose application will solve problems within that domain. Engineering is a practical domain concerned with construction and the techniques of engineering analysis, design and execution are the means by which engineering outcomes (constructions) are achieved.[6]

In this respect, medicine is obviously a practical domain concerned with health whose desired outcomes are the protection and improvement of health. The techniques of medicine are those in which medical practitioners are trained, from diagnosis to prescribed care to serious intervention. In the ordinary case, medical problems are solved by the application of medical techniques. Problems in medical ethics often have the form, 'Can we solve this medical problem using these techniques?' For instance, can we secure this child's long-term health by growth attenuation therapy? Or, can we treat this patient's body dysmorphic disorder by surgical amputation of a limb? Problems in medical ethics with this form are problems concerning which actions (applications of techniques) are permissible for achieving outcomes in health.

Consequentialism seems a natural fit for practical problems because it is concerned with the outcomes of actions. I take consequentialism to be an ethical theory whose signature tenet is the evaluation of actions solely according to their outcomes.[7] Prospectively, someone reasoning from consequentialist ethical principles should evaluate actions according to their expected outcomes. For example, to determine to which charity I should give, I should consider which will use my contribution to produce the best outcome for those the charity helps. Retrospectively, an action should be evaluated in consequentialist terms according to its outcome. For example, I can conclude my charitable contribution was ethically inferior to one I could have made if the same contribution to a different charity would have produced a better outcome, for example, people helped more effectively.

There are many variants of consequentialism. Some evaluate actions and their outcomes by their intended versus actual outcomes. Some evaluate actions according to their conformance to rules or motives, each of which is approved by its tendency to conduce to good outcomes. It is essential to a consequentialist ethical outlook that one is committed to using principles of ethical reasoning in which evaluative assessments are ultimately of outcomes, real or imagined, effected by the actions of moral subjects. At any rate, in my use of 'consequentialism' below, this will be the defining character referred to by the term.

The first reason consequentialism seems a natural fit for medical ethics is that they share a concern with evaluating the outcomes of actions. That is, each embodies methods for evaluating solutions to practical problems.

The second reason consequentialism seems a natural fit is that it is easily able to evaluate outcomes in which people are considered as a population or aggregate. For instance, a notorious consequentialist principle is maximizing the greatest happiness for the greatest number. The principle could have been used in the examples concerning charitable contributions above to make more precise the basis for evaluating the outcome of one contribution over another, that is, contribute to the charity that will help the greatest number to the greatest extent.

Consequentialists, committed to the evaluation of actions by their outcomes, are ultimately committed to evaluations of states of affairs. For it is states of affairs that are the outcomes of the actions of moral subjects. The *basis* for the evaluation of states of affairs is not essential to an outlook being consequentialist. One consequentialist may evaluate states of affairs by the happiness of those constituting the states of affairs, another by the exemplification of the virtues of those constituting the state of affairs. What is essential is (i) that each has a basis for such evaluations and (ii) that such evaluations are in turn the basis for ethical assessments of actions – or what comes to the same thing, the evaluation of rules for or motives to action by the extent to which each conduces to states of affairs that would be assessed as better on the basis of (i).

The important point is that consequentialist outlooks take as their ethical focus – the object of moral consideration – states of affairs, considered as the outcomes of potential actions. Medical ethics is well-acquainted with problems in which the foci are states of affairs constituted by aggregates of people, that is, populations. Triage is a well-known technique for getting the best outcome overall for a population of injured. Medical quarantine is a policy that seeks a state of affairs for one population by placing preventive restrictions on another population. Vaccination policies are similar. The allocation of scarce medical resources is a situation in which different populations of need must be weighed against each other.

In these cases, the people comprising the populations are not considered as individual people, but rather as populations constituting states of affairs. The outcomes sought from these policies are defined as outcomes for a population, for example, increased survival rates, reduced morbidity, increased aggregate health outcomes. This way of thinking is common in medical policy-making, formulating codes of medical ethics, as well as cases of the kinds described above. Consequentialism is an ethical outlook that accommodates and complements this kind of thinking because of its focus on outcomes conceived as states of affairs.

There are then two good reasons for thinking that medical ethics and consequentialism go together well and this explains why consequentialist thinking features often in discussions of medical ethics. Deontological ethical outlooks, by contrast, do not seem so accommodating. By a deontological ethical outlook I shall understand an ethical outlook whose focus is one's duties. In a deontological outlook, an action is correct when it is in accord with one's duties. Deontology too comes in many variants. For instance some vary by the variety, origins or kinds of duties they acknowledge; some vary by whether accord with duty must be absolute; others by whether duties are a species of another ethical genus like values.

Deontological theories have enough in common though, to bring out their conflict with those features of consequentialism that make consequentialism seem agreeable for medical ethics. Deontology is not indifferent to consequence, because the consideration of the likely outcomes of actions is important for considering which are in accord with one's duties.

However, whereas consequentialist thinking may be used to select from among actions, any of which is a solution to a practical problem, deontological considerations are as apt to create practical problems as to solve them. A consequentialist can always choose one solution to a problem, indeed he ought to select the solution with the best outcome, even if that outcome is overall a negative one. That is, he can always make the best of a bad situation. However, if no solution to a problem is in accord with (some) duties, then a deontologist cannot choose any. He cannot always make the best of a bad situation. For instance, for some deontological outlooks, euthanasia is not permissible even if it would avoid certain, slow, painful death.

Deontology is not practical in the sense described above. It would not be entirely unfair to say that deontology is concerned to identify constraints in solving problems rather than selecting solutions. For this reason, it can create new practical problems, for example, by barring solutions to an otherwise readily soluble problem. A deontologist may believe that the best outcome would come from deceiving a patient and making him believe that he has most reason to do so, but yet believe that ethically he must not.

Second, deontological outlooks are typically resistant to considering people as constituents of aggregates, for reasons that apply variously. First, individual people are the primary locus of the demands of duty, for example, a duty to aid or of non-interference. Second, in hierarchies of duties, those duties owed to individual people (including oneself) are typically at the top of the hierarchy. Third, even when one's duty is owed because someone falls under a group or within a population – for example, one's neighbours – an action must accord with the duty owed to him because he is a neighbour, not because of a duty owed to a population of which he is one constituent. That is, he is considered as an individual, even though the duties owed to him are identified in part by reference to the groups he part-constitutes.

In this sketch of a comparison several things are evident. Deontology is not well suited to ethical challenges conceived as practical problems, unlike consequentialism. Deontology is typically resistant to treating people in aggregate, unlike consequentialism. For these reasons, deontology seems an inferior match for medical ethics compared to consequentialism. Moreover, it should be clear why the analysis of a medical ethical challenge can differ to the extent of contrariety depending on whether the analysis is from a consequentialist or deontological outlook. For the difference of outlook is not solely between the weight accorded to one or more values, but is between what is morally salient to the analysis of the situation. One considers outcomes, the other considers duties. It could seem that they might not even agree on the identity or character of the challenge.

Two Arguments

I have sought to show that consequentialism is a presumptive best fit for medical ethics. I suggest this is one reason for its appeal. I have also sought to elaborate the importance accorded to autonomy in some domains of medical ethics, viz. those concerning quality of life. I offer below two arguments to the effect that consequentialist outlooks cannot take account of autonomy. This is preliminary to my concluding that this dialectical outcome nullifies the presumptive appeal of consequentialist thinking for medical ethics.

The first argument begins from the observation that autonomy or its exercise cannot be the intended outcome of an action. The second argument is that consequentialism is at its roots indifferent to the aetiology of states of affairs and is therefore indifferent to whether states of affairs are effected autonomously.

Autonomy is not a state of affairs, therefore it can make no sense to say that it is the intended or actual outcome of an action. Autonomous action – the expression of autonomy in action – can be a state of affairs. When someone acts autonomously, they are part of a state of affairs in which there is autonomous action, namely that someone's action. However, this cannot be the intended outcome of an action for the subject or object of the action.

A moral subject cannot act with the intention of acting autonomously, unless the word is taken with existentialist overtones connoting authenticity, the absence of bad faith, etc. Autonomy is, of itself, empty as an action. By this I mean that it always makes sense to ask what the object of an action is, even when one knows that the acting subject is acting autonomously. A clue is in the fact that we use 'autonomy' and its cognates linguistically to modify something: adverbially, 'He acted autonomously when taking the stand'; as an adjective, 'Suicide is never an autonomous action'; or in a prepositional clause, 'His defiance was an expression of his autonomy'. Another way to express the point is that autonomous action is not itself a doing (an action) but is just a *way* of doing. It is easy to see the same point in an analogy with acting quickly. It is not clear *what* was done when one knows that someone acted quickly, though one has some idea *how* it was done. Therefore, absent context, when one says they intend to act autonomously, it is always appropriate to ask, 'To do what?'

If I am right that autonomy is as empty as an action, I conclude that autonomy itself cannot figure among the actions whose outcomes a consequentialist is concerned to consider because it is no action. Similarly, the choice between two actions, one done autonomously and the other not, is also, as a choice, empty. For it is not possible to choose a non-autonomous action. We could allow that it is possible to act non-autonomously, for instance when one is hypnotized or drugged. It is not possible to choose to act non-autonomously because choosing that action is just the expression of one's autonomy. Therefore, a putatively non-autonomous action is transmuted into an autonomous one, by it being chosen, that is, by the exercise of autonomy. In this way, a prisoner can assert his dignity by autonomously choosing what he would in any case be forced to do. As another example, psychotherapy is successful when the patient is able to do autonomously what he in any case had to do, for example, admit his self-deception.

These considerations show that with regard to the subject who acts, it cannot be his autonomy or its expression in his actions which is among the outcomes he evaluates in a consequentialist outlook. It is somewhat easier to see why someone else's autonomy cannot be the object of one's action, not directly at least. An action whose intended outcome is to determine the action of another person is *ipso facto* one that is counter to the other person's autonomy. For the outcome of the subject's action, if successful, will be an action by a person (the action's object) that is not autonomous. How could it be an autonomous action when it was *determined* by another, that is, is other-determined? I do not make someone's action autonomous by drugging them or deceiving them into doing it – even if they would have done it anyway. No doubt there may be shades of grey, such as whether Othello's killing of Desdemona was autonomous. The importance of clarifying such a case lies in establishing Othello's moral responsibility. However that turns out, it is clear that Iago was not acting in favour of autonomy by his exploitation of Othello's insecurities.

The conclusion is that, formally, consequentialism is blind to autonomy when reasoning about which action is best, therefore it cannot urge or oblige the selection of actions and outcomes based on differences in autonomy. Since autonomy cannot figure among the consequences (outcomes) of an action, it can have no normative impact in guiding action within a consequentialist outlook. Roughly, consequentialists cannot value autonomy prospectively.

I advertised a second, more general, problem for taking account of autonomy within a consequentialist outlook. The roots of the problem are latent in the discussion of the first argument. There, it was clear that autonomy did not contribute to *what* was effected by an action, but rather *how* the action effected its outcome. However, consequentialism, as is evident from the name, is an ethical outlook concerned with what an action effects – its consequences – not how it effects it. Therefore, again, a consequentialist outlook is blind to autonomy because it is indifferent to outcomes produced autonomously and those produced non-autonomously. Roughly, consequentialists cannot value autonomy retrospectively.

To be clear, consequentialism is indifferent to outcomes produced autonomously or not, because the outcomes of states of affairs are indistinguishable on the basis of autonomy since, as shown above, autonomy is not part of a state of affairs. It will not do to reply that an action done autonomously will have a different outcome to one done non-autonomously. First, if the outcomes were indeed different then one would *not* be choosing between them solely on their differences in autonomy. The choice would be on the basis of the differing consequences, just as consequentialism requires. Second, consequentialism's indifference to autonomy is evident when we consider that any autonomous action's outcome can be conceived as the outcome of a non-autonomous action. In which case, there is no basis in a consequentialist outlook to favour one action over the other. For example, for any action done autonomously – such as taking one's medication – a non-autonomous counterpart can always be conceived, e.g. having been deceived into taking the medication. The outcomes are the same, viz. the medication is taken. Absent any difference in outcome, there is no consequentialist reason for preferring one to another.

We can sketch why this is a feature of the consequentialist outlook. For a consequentialist, the loci of value are in states of affairs. That is, what is good in the world is not how people conduct themselves *per se*, but the states of affairs to which people give rise by their actions. To put it another way, for a consequentialist, the priority, at least in the order of specification, is the good (the what) before the right (the how). Put in a parallel formulation, the priority for a consequentialist is a state of affairs (the what) before its aetiology (how it came to be). So it is not surprising that consequentialism is at its roots indifferent to the aetiology of states of affairs. The aetiology of a state of affairs, where it concerns moral subjects, will arise within this outlook as a secondary question concerning moral responsibility, viz. who caused this state of affairs?[8]

Objections

I turn to objections to my arguments that consequentialism is blind to autonomy.

The first objection is that we often do act so as to promote autonomy. For instance, parents give children opportunities to act autonomously, when allowing them choice or other liberties. A doctor who gives a patient relevant information concerning courses of treatment frees the patient from acting in ignorance. So it is mistaken to suppose that consequentialists are blind to autonomy when evaluating actions.

Certainly we can differentiate those actions that promote autonomy. However, these actions can at most make autonomy more *likely*. None has as its outcome that autonomy will be exercised.Therefore, none is an action that could be valued more because its outcome includes an *exercise* of autonomy. Rather one could value an outcome over another because it makes *possible* the exercise of autonomy. The argument that consequentialism cannot value the exercise of autonomy is therefore not addressed by this objection. At best, the value of autonomy in a consequentialist outlook is *indirect*.

A different expression of this point is that there is no action by which someone becomes autonomous who was not already autonomous. Autonomy is not something someone can bestow. A drug can be removed from the water, subliminal messaging from the airwaves, or a dictator from power. In each case we can assert that a person or people is now autonomous. However, we have not thereby made them autonomous, we solely removed an obstacle to exercising the autonomy they already had. If right, then we cannot act to create autonomy as an outcome.

A second objection is that if states of affairs can have a character that is not present in the individual entities in the state of affairs, why cannot autonomy be in a state of affairs? For instance, a state of affairs can be just, that is, justice is so-to-speak present in the state of affairs. Yet, no element is itself justice. Justice is in a state of affairs, why not autonomy?

Justice is a relational property amongst elements in a state of affairs, e.g. the distribution of resources in a society is just, perhaps, according to the relations between the resources and the members of the society.[9] However, there is no analogy with autonomy. I noted above that one cannot bestow autonomy. So no action can add autonomy, as one can add resources, to a state of affairs. Moreover, the argument in the previous section against the possibility of acting to determine another's action as autonomous, entails that *no* action can add a relationship of autonomy between an actor and his action, as one can add the relationship of ownership between resources and persons. In short, actions can alter the distribution of resources, but there is no parallel for action. I suggest this dis-analogy will be true for any relational property in a state of affairs. The objection is therefore ineffective, because it is not analogous.

Motive consequentialism enables a third objection. Motive consequentialism is a form of indirect consequentialism in which actions are selected not for their consequences, but by whether they are motivated by motives that conduce to better states of affairs.[10] For instance, actions motivated by kindness, plausibly conduce to better states of affairs, than those motivated by self-interest. That is, generally, kind actions produce better states of affairs than self-interested actions. In this consequentialist outlook, an action is correct, if it is motivated by better motives than others. The objection is that we fix the normative blindness of consequentialism to autonomy by making autonomy one of the motives we consider in evaluating actions.

Autonomy is not a motive, however. So the objection is misconceived. However, even if autonomy were a motive, there is no reason to think that autonomy conduces to better (or worse) states of affairs. The millennia-old problem of evil – viz. that we may with our free will do evil as easily as good – is surely adequate testimony that autonomy by itself does not conduce to good. Unlike with a kind action, when I know an action was autonomous, I know nothing of its ethical character. Therefore, the objection, misconceived from the start, fails.

The fourth objection is the strongest and most illuminating of the consequentialist outlook and its normative indifference to autonomy. Several arguments have shown that states of affairs with autonomous actions cannot be conceived as the outcomes of actions. However, the expression or exercise of autonomy is not restricted to action. We can distinguish preferences and desires as being autonomous or not (i.e. heteronomous), as we distinguish those that we call true or false. For instance, the desires of someone in thrall to dogma may not be his own but another's; or the preferences of someone who is ill may be shaped by his despair and are in this sense not his true preferences. The distinctions may be difficult, but that there is such a distinction – sometimes well-founded – is not in doubt.

We can imagine a consequentialist outlook in which states of affairs are better if more autonomous desires and preferences are satisfied. So given two states of affairs with superficially identical desires and preferences, save that in one the desires and preferences are autonomous (self-determined) and in another they are not, this consequentialist evaluates the 'autonomous state of affairs' as better. In this way, this consequentialist is able to give normative weight to the expression or exercise of autonomy.

Is this is an intelligible account of better states of affairs, where they are better just because more autonomous desires and preferences are satisfied? It is not incoherent, but as an account of ethical evaluation it seems curiously neutral: Is *any* desire preferred, if autonomous? Perhaps these desires and preferences are to be understood as the constituents of individual conceptions of happiness.

I grant that the conception is possible and that it would give some normative weight to autonomy within a consequentialist outlook. To that extent, the objection succeeds. However, if this is the best that can be done it reveals how a person is conceived through the consequentialist's lens of action as effecting states of affairs. On the view sketched, people – human beings – are to be understood as bundles of unsatisfied desires and preferences. New states of affairs affect them insofar as some of their preferences or desires are satisfied and new ones are created. As it were, the practical problem faced by a decision-maker is which techniques to employ to satisfy the preferences and desires of those within the scope of the states of affairs that may be effected. Treating people in aggregate is easy because doing so is a matter of treating their preferences and desires in aggregate. Indeed, each person is himself a localized state of affairs – constituted by preferences and desires – ready for aggregation.

Once people are considered in this way, two things become clear. First, it does not matter when evaluating actions whether preferences and desires are satisfied by the person whose preferences and desires they are, only that they are satisfied. So insofar as valuing autonomy requires recognizing others as the motive force in their lives – as I suggested above – even this refined consequentialism remains normatively blind to this aspect of autonomy.[11] This is a consequence of its root indifference to the aetiology of states of affairs. What matters is which preferences and desires are satisfied, not how or by whom. For example, treatment by dissociative drugs would be as good as treatment without, if the outcomes are the same.

Second, indifference to *how* someone's preferences and desires are satisfied is an aspect of indifference to other moral responses bearing on autonomy. For example, a doctor responding with pity to someone's condition will certainly act differently than responding without pity. Yet recognizing someone as pitiable does not require any dissent from an assessment of which are the patient's preferences or desires. As it were, for the consequentialist, if pitying is not related to an autonomous preference or desire, it is of no normative import, that is, no ethical import. Pity is especially problematic, since autonomous pity would be self-pity, which is different again from pity and probably not a desire to satisfy. So consequentialists, by indifference to aetiology, are blind to more than autonomy.

Acting mercifully in which one acts contrary to what is normatively indicated – in this case autonomous preferences and desires – is another problematic case of an ethical response to which the consequentialist is blind. Ethical responses like these are ones I characterized in the Introduction as forms of attention, but not the attention we give to a practical problem. A response to a practical problem is a search for a solution. But responses of pity, mercy and respect are not solution-seeking responses because the responses need make no difference to which preferences or desires are satisfied, indeed they can make things worse in these terms. The ways in which they can make the situation worse, in the practical terms of a consequentialist, can be exactly those that implicate autonomy. For instance, out of respect, the best thing to do is to allow a disabled person to do things for himself, even though they could be done more effectively by someone else. For another example, out of pity for someone's descent into addiction, one may collude in his self-deceptive fictions, even though this will prolong his recovery. These are ethical responses not only because they are expressions of the value of autonomy, but because each also expresses a further ethical value: for pity it is fellowship; for respect, humility; for mercy, compassion.

Therefore, while I have allowed that a particular consequentialist outlook can give normative weight to autonomy, it is an attenuated sense of autonomy that is severed from the ethical responses by which we express the *value* of autonomy. The ordinary expressions of the value of autonomy are of course those which I have suggested by assumption are the most important in the confrontation between doctor and patient. They are also the responses that illuminate the relationship between autonomy and allied concepts like dignity, authority, and freedom.

Conclusions

I have sought to show that consequentialism, contrary to appearances, is not suited to medical ethics, if autonomy is taken as a central value in medical practice. The reason it is ill-suited as an ethical outlook is that it is normatively blind to autonomy. If the consequentialist outlook is gerrymandered to give priority to one's expression of autonomy, the value of autonomy therein is attenuated. Indeed, structural features of consequentialism mean that it cannot accommodate several desirable expressions of the value of autonomy, that is, pity, respect and mercy. If I am right, then in medical ethical debates by presumption we ought to preclude introducing considerations from a consequentialist ethical outlook.

I have not argued that autonomy is central to ethical medical practice, rather I have assumed that it is; by its centrality in recent debates, medical education, promulgated codes of ethics for medical practitioners. That is one limit of my argument.

I have argued for a conception of autonomy that is wider than that which solely concerns consent and the acknowledgement of someone's authority over their body. Rather, I have argued that autonomy is a concept that encompasses someone's making his life his own by being the motivating force within it, where this means both conceiving his course and realizing that course – to the extent he can. The necessity to do so arises from the lack of an authority – legitimate or derived from expertise – on a good life. Paying attention to someone, taking him seriously, respecting his autonomy requires attention, seriousness and respect for him as the author of his life story and the perspective that story expresses.

A further, significant limit of my argument then is that it is most cogent when addressing this wider notion of autonomy. Where autonomy is not at issue or where the notion of autonomy at issue is that concerned solely with consent, then the dialectical burden on the consequentialist should be lifted. Several examples illustrate this limitation. The ethical status of stem cells is one example with no implication for autonomy. The distribution of scarce medical resources is another with no implications for autonomy, since the overriding priorities of justice or fairness requires that people are treated homogeneously without regard to their differing conceptions of life. Whether treatment should be compulsory is an ethical challenge that *can* arise with implications for autonomy solely in the narrow sense of consent.

Notwithstanding the challenges that fall into the category excluded from the force of my intended conclusion, there is still an expansive category where the burden of proof should be against introducing a consequentialist outlook. Euthanasia, rights to die, options to die and similar end-of-life and quality-of-life ethical challenges are saturated with this wider notion of autonomy. Compulsory treatment challenges can arise so as to implicate this wider notion of autonomy too. For instance, someone with a terminal illness can refuse treatment because they do not want their last months disfigured by the interventions of therapy or palliative care. Issues arising from those who are unable to express their autonomy – owing to youth or incapacity – will also implicate, however hypothetically, this wider notion of the life they would or should seek.

This is so far not to win a ready response to these problems. For autonomy is not the only ethical value to which doctors owe fidelity. After all, medical practitioners are not a *de facto* cash and carry, where any expression of autonomy is delivered up to a would-be patient at his request. There must be limits to autonomy or, if not limits, balancing considerations, such as when the patient is the origin of the illness. Consider the patient who is enamoured of the Pro-Ana movement that advocates anorexia as an alternative lifestyle choice. Does it make sense to talk of successful *outcomes* for this patient without paying attention to his autonomy – beyond consent – while being responsive to the other ethical demands his situation makes on us? I suggest it does not. More, I have argued that if it does not, then we should be wary of assessing our actions in terms of outcomes, as the consequentialist would urge.

Chapter 9

Respecting Patients' Religious Beliefs

David Albert Jones

Non-Overlapping Magisteria

What is the relevance of the fact that a patient may profess a religious belief and may seek to live according to that belief to the ethical practice of medicine? In what way, if at all, should a medical professional 'respect' the patient's religious belief?

One possible reaction to this question is to claim that religious belief is of no relevance to ethical medical practice. In the wake of the atrocities committed by doctors in Nazi Germany, the World Medical Association recommitted itself to ethical medicine through a re-statement of the Hippocratic Oath: The Declaration of Geneva 1948 (Jones 2006). The context of this statement was crimes against humanity and, in particular, crimes against the Jewish people, who comprise both a religion and an ethnic group. So it is unsurprising that the Declaration included an explicit rejection of discrimination based on religion or race: 'I will not permit considerations of religion, nationality, race, party politics, or social standing to intervene between my duty and my patient'. The revisions of the Declaration in 1994 and 2005 expand the list of prohibited forms of discrimination, but still include reference to 'creed' and 'ethnic origin'.

The Declaration opposes all forms of discrimination that 'intervene' between the doctor and his or her duty to the patient. On the face of it, this seems to imply that religion or creed is a factor to which medicine should be blind. Treatment decisions should be based on medical indications and this applies equally irrespective of the patient's religion.

To hold this would not be to deny that religion is a valuable or worthwhile activity, nor that religion might occasionally motivate harmful or unhealthy behaviour. Rather, it would simply be to assert that the realm of medicine is separate from and independent of religion. The best way for the doctor to respect the patient's religion is, on this view, to ignore this aspect entirely. It is not the doctor's business. The doctor is concerned for the body while religion attends to the soul. There may or may not be a soul and religion may or may not be a waste of time, but in any case the proper focus of religion is with matters other than the physical health of the body.

Admittedly physical and mental ill health, the approach of death, and the fact of bereavement are all occasions of spiritual need. Therefore, there is certainly a role for religious ministers, chaplains or others to attend to the spiritual needs of people who are ill. Hospitals may employ chaplains just as the military and the prison service employ chaplains, in recognition that in times of stress people have personal, existential, or spiritual needs. However, attending to this aspect of the human person is essentially separate from the aims and methods of medicine: the hospital chaplain is no more a healthcare worker than the prison chaplain is a jailor or the army chaplain a combatant. He or she may work with but also stand apart from the healthcare team.

It was the agnostic Jewish biologist Stephen J Gould who popularized the term 'nonoverlapping magisteria' to express the view that religion and science answer different questions (Gould 1997). Their explanations are not of the same order and hence, at least in general, they are not in competition or conflict. Gould notes that what he calls the oxymoron of 'creation science' is a localized feature of Protestantism in the United States (and indeed only one form of Protestantism). Scientific theories about the origin of species by means of natural selection were simply not viewed as a problem by mainstream Jewish and Catholic religious authorities, as they were accustomed to deal with texts in a sophisticated manner, and did not regard the opening chapters of Genesis as written in the same genre as descriptions in the natural sciences.

However, this irenic vision, even if it can be applied to religion and the natural sciences (and even here it seems that there may sometimes be overlap), is difficult to apply to medicine. For the relationship of theology to the natural sciences is primarily theoretic, and in this context it is quite possible to maintain that they are diverse bodies of knowledge which often do not relate directly to one another. In contrast, medicine is not solely a body of theoretical knowledge but is also a set of practices informed by knowledge and skill.

The concern about a possible tension between medicine and religion is less at the level of explanation and more about impact on practice. When thinking, in retrospect about whether a person recovers because of a medical intervention or as an answer to prayer, there is certainly room to suggest that it could be both. So also a religious person might see an episode of mental ill health as an attack by evil spirits, but this is not necessarily a problem looking back. It becomes potentially problematic in relation to medicine precisely as a practice, if for example it inhibits the patients from accepting medical treatment or is the basis of requests for inappropriate treatment.

As medicine is practical it is therefore forced to interact with the practical effects of religion as these have an impact on delivering healthcare. And clearly religion can affect the practical decision-making of patients.

The Warfare of Science with Theology

The Secular Medical Forum, which exists to oppose 'religious influences in medicine where these affect the manner in which medical practice is performed' (2009), gives several examples of the de facto influence of religion in medical practice. The main areas of conflict listed on the website are 'Abortion', 'Advance Decisions', 'Conscientious Objections', 'Hospital Chaplains', 'HIV/AIDS', 'Physician-Assisted Suicide', 'Religious Surgery on Children' (i.e. circumcision), 'Sex Education' and 'Stem Cell Research'. It is noticeable that most of these examples concern a moral outlook rather than religion *per se* and there is no mention of the hackneyed example of Jehovah's Witnesses refusing blood transfusions. This may be because the moral outlook of the SMF is libertarian: 'pro-choice' including the choice to die by refusing treatment. What the SMF are most concerned about is that religious doctors may refuse to comply with the wishes of patients, for example because of conscientious objection.

Another highly contentious area of concern to anti-religious campaigners is the religious practice of exorcism to 'expel demons' from people with mental health problems. Even the suggestion that exorcism might be beneficial to some patients is regarded by some secular critics as sufficient to question a doctor's fitness to practice (see, for example, the blog *Religion versus medicine* (2010)).[1] As religion clearly has an impact on the practice of medicine it seems reasonable to begin by examining the claim that religion has a real but a 'grotesque influence on medicine and health' (*Religion versus medicine* (2010)). In the words of the celebrated atheist Richard Dawkins, 'I think a case can be made that *faith* is one of the world's great evils, comparable to the smallpox virus but harder to eradicate' (Dawkins 1997),

Before turning to evidence of the conflict between medicine and religion from history and from contemporary practice, it is helpful to examine an *a priori* argument for the same conclusion. It is widely accepted that the successes of modern medicine are due to progress in scientific understanding of human biology. Medicine thus presents itself as a practical application of scientific knowledge. In contrast religion, by its own admission, is based on faith and/or on traditional practice. If rationality is exemplified by the rigour of scientific medicine then religion cannot but appear less than rational. However, if religion is an irrational force in culture and society it will only by accident agree with what is rational and reasonable. It should therefore be regarded with the utmost suspicion and confined to areas of private life which cannot adversely affect the lives of others.

It is worth setting out this argument explicitly as it seems to underlie the way that apparent conflicts are interpreted as conflicts about the natural causes of health and disease. Where there is dispute about the causes or effects of disease or medicine these are indeed normally best resolved by appeal to scientific methods. However a cursory review of the areas of conflict identified by the Secular Medical Forum shows a preponderance of ethical questions – abortion, euthanasia, stem cell research – and ethical questions cannot be resolved by scientific research except where there is already common agreement about ethical principles. Whatever the correct interpretation of David Hume's dictum that one cannot deduce an 'ought' from an 'is', it is clear that natural science on its own does not provide a basis for moral decision-making. *Pace* Hume, this does not show that reason plays little role in morality. Both reason and argument play an important role in morality, but this is because the method of the natural sciences is not the only expression of human reason. Not only critical moral reflection but theology, philosophy and indeed all the humanities (politics, history, literary criticism) embody forms of rationality and argument distinct from and irreducible to the methods of the natural sciences.

The idea that religion can be dismissed in advance as irrational, and only helpful by accident, may be based on the belief that there is no God. However, the question of whether or not there is a God, and thus whether all religious beliefs are based on a falsehood, is not itself a scientific question (this is indeed Gould's central point). It belongs rather to philosophy or 'natural theology'. Atheism is itself a theological position (the denial of certain theological assertions). Atheism constitutes a worldview and competes with other theological worldviews.

The attempt to exclude religious influences on healthcare can thus be seen as an attempt to impose one theology, that of atheism, upon the diversity of religious beliefs. However, there are no *a priori* grounds for privileging atheism within healthcare. An atheist may argue that atheism should be the default theological position in the absence of compelling evidence or cogent argument for God's existence, but this assertion is clearly self-serving. Given the ubiquity of religion in every age and in every culture it is not obvious that the denial of all religion should be the default position. Nevertheless, if there is no *a priori* case for atheism there may still be an atheist case to be made, for example, using evidence from history that religious belief has been more of a hindrance than a help to medicine.

The classic statement of this argument is found in AD White's book *The Warfare of Science with Theology in Christendom* (1896), itself influenced by JD Williams' *History of the Conflict between Religion and Science* (1874). White devotes an entire chapter to the allegedly malign effects of religion on medical progress. This chapter is worth examining because it remains influential. Not only is it available in its entirety on the internet but examples from this chapter have been reiterated in public debate as recently as 2005. One example may suffice to give a flavour of the chapter.

> In 1847, James Young Simpson, a Scotch physician, who afterward rose to the highest eminence in his profession, having advocated the use of anaesthetics in obstetrical cases, was immediately met by a storm of opposition ... From pulpit after pulpit Simpson's use of chloroform was denounced as impious and contrary to Holy Writ; texts were cited abundantly, the ordinary declaration being that to use chloroform was 'to avoid one part of the primeval curse on woman.' (White 1896 pp. 62–63)

This example has been much quoted, recently for example by the pro-euthanasia theologian Paul Badham (2005). However, the evidence for this 'storm of opposition' is limited to a pamphlet written by Simpson in which he defends his practice against real or imagined critics. In fact no Christian denomination, no Christian tract, no prominent Churchman opposed the development of anaesthetic (Farr 1983). The idea of significant Christian opposition to anaesthetics in childbirth seems to be a myth based on a *Christian* tract defending the innovation. Since the 1960s it has been widely recognized that the thesis of a generic and repeated 'conflict' of science and religion is inadequate to the historical data and should be understood rather as a particular expression of late nineteenth century historiography (Brooke 1991, Ferngren 2002). It is a classic case of eisegesis, historians reading into texts and events a significance that these did not carry in their original context.

The idea of a mythic conflict of medicine and religion is further undermined by the abundant evidence of the positive effects of religion on the development of healthcare. This is admitted even by White:

> This spirit [of Jesus of Nazareth] then poured into the world, flowed down through the ages, promoting self-sacrifice for the sick and wretched.

> Through all those succeeding centuries, even through the rudest, hospitals and infirmaries sprang up along this blessed stream. Of these were the Eastern establishments for the cure of the sick at the earliest Christian periods, the Infirmary of Monte Cassino and the Hotel-Dieu at Lyons in the sixth century, the Hotel-Dieu at Paris in the seventh, and the myriad refuges for the sick and suffering which sprang up in every part of Europe during the following centuries (White 1896 p. 3).

White also comments positively on the contribution that Jewish and Islamic physicians and medical schools made to the progress of medicine. Thus even White, in a highly polemical work devoted to demonstrating the existence of an essential conflict between science and religion cannot deny that religion has also had significant beneficial effects (see for example Risse 1999, Ferngren 2009, Clark 2001). This leads naturally to the question of whether religion might continue to have a beneficial effect in a modern context, and not only on healthcare but directly on health outcomes.

Is Religion Good for Your Health?

In contrast to those who see religious belief as a kind of pathology, detrimental both to health and to medical practice, there are others who have argued vigorously that religious practice is beneficial for health. Perhaps the most substantial presentation of this case is that of Harold G. Koenig whose magisterial *Medicine, Religion, and Health: Where Science and Spirituality Meet* (2008) gathers evidence from a great range of countries and medical disciplines. Koenig argues that religion has measurable health benefits in helping patients cope positively with illnesses and diagnoses. In arguing that religious belief has a positive effect on mental health Koenig is following a line of argument that is at least as old as Jung. It is true that many schools of psychology (by no means limited to Freudians) have regarded religious belief as an impediment to maturity and mental health. In an area where there is no agreed methodology and there is fierce antagonism between different schools of thought, Koenig seeks to bring empirical evidence of health benefit, and not only to mental health but also physical health.

Levin (1994) has argued that correlations between religion and health of the kind identified by Koenig are not directly causal but are mediated by other factors such as income, social stability and lifestyle. It is indeed notoriously difficult to establish causal relations in matters of well-being and this certainly requires more than positive statistical correlations. Nevertheless, if positive correlations are mediated by, for example, lifestyle choices, then this causal mechanism is itself an expression of religion. It is not only through internal psychological or spiritual mechanisms that religion makes its influence felt, for religion is a social phenomenon. This can also be illustrated by the evidence supplied by Neeleman *et al* (1997) that there is an inverse correlation between individual religious belief and suicide, and that in men (but for some reason not in women) suicide is also inhibited by the strength of religion in the culture as a whole. Neeleman argues that the predominant mechanism of this suppression is in shaping attitudes about what is acceptable: 'exposure to a religious environment may protect against suicide by reducing its acceptability' (1997 p. 1165).

To attribute a positive effect of religion on health is not therefore to accept the truth claims of any specific religion or to posit a supernatural causal mechanism. Research on the general effect of religion on health should not be confused with experiments aiming to demonstrate the efficacy or inefficacy of petitionary prayer. Still more should it be distinguished from claims that a particular healing event is 'miraculous' in the sense of defying medical explanation. Many religious traditions include both petitionary prayer and the possibility of miracles. However we see this, the category of 'miraculous healing' is narrower and more specific than healing as an answer to prayer and the category of 'answered prayer' is itself narrower than the category of health benefit. Religion may be beneficial for health for quite mundane reasons.

A further distinction which can be made in this context is between religion and spirituality. While religion is defined by practice and by assent to statements of belief, spirituality is essentially concerned with one's personal response to the existential realities of life and death. Several scholars have sought to draw up a definition of spirituality independent of religious practice and belief; for example Frey defines spirituality as 'a congruent, meaningful life scheme and high functional self-efficacy beliefs that synergistically promote personal agency' (Frey *et al.* 2005 p. 561). This definition supports a measure of spiritual well-being: Spirituality Index of Well-Being (SIWB),according to Frey, is an accurate predictor of self-rated good health (p. 563, see also Katerndahl 2008). Those who define spirituality in this way distinguish it from religiosity and frequently claim that it is spiritual well-being that is a determinant of health and not religion per se. The realm of spirituality understood in this way is a generic aspect of the human being, common to people of all religions and none. In this way spiritual well-being can be thought of as an aspect of complete well-being in line with the World Health Organisation definition of health. In 1946 the WHO defined health as 'a state of complete physical, mental and social well-being and not merely the absence of disease or infirmity'. As the WHO introduced a wide definition of health which in principle could be extended to spiritual well-being, so Dame Cecily Saunders, pioneer in the discipline of palliative care, introduced a wide definition of 'total pain' that included the physical, emotional, social, and (explicitly) the spiritual dimensions of distress (Richmond 2005). If medical professionals are to address the pain of the patient they must therefore be aware of not only physical pain or well-being but also spiritual pain or well-being.

The language of 'spirituality', 'spiritual well-being', 'spiritual pain' and 'spiritual care' has brought religion into the ambit of healthcare and from a religious perspective this may seem a positive thing. Nevertheless, this move has long been resisted by some religious believers. For example, while Jung wished to put forward a positive account of religion (in contrast to Freud), the theological dialogue between Jung and the Dominican friar Victor White eventually broke down (White 1960, Lammers & Cunningham 2007, Weldon 2007). White could not accept Jung's reinterpretation of Christian language. Even if Christianity is often beneficial for mental health, this nevertheless is not the aim or focus of Christianity. Theology is not reducible to psychology. The language of 'sin' and 'grace', of 'heaven' and 'hell', of 'creation' and 'redemption' are not taken by theologians to refer only to states of consciousness. While the idea of God exists in the mind of the believer and may positively influence his or her psychology, Theology is concerned first and foremost not with this influence but with God as the creator outside the mind. If there is no God then Theology is based on a false premise. Indeed, White points out that in some cases Christianity may require actions that are a burden to mental health and which may have an adverse effect on the believer's subjective experience of well-being. This should be expected because mental health is not the only or the highest good and, from a Christian perspective, the search for mental health should not be set up as a religion (on a similar point see Sloan *et al.* 2000).

It is also worthy of note that the very broad WHO definition of health has been criticized by some religious bioethicists. Luke Gormally, for example, has argued that the WHO definition is too wide as it allows medical technology to be applied to social goals beyond the good of physical health (Gormally 1997). This gives an apparent justification for practices such as abortion, sterilization and gender re-assignment. It is noteworthy that in England, Wales and Scotland, the supposed legal justification for abortion is as a health benefit to the expectant mother. While such practices are contrary to the traditional ethic of medicine, as expressed, for example, in the Hippocratic Oath (Jones 2006), they are now advocated on the basis of an expanded definition of health.

Gormally's argument applies even more strongly to a definition of healthcare that is wide enough to include spirituality. This is not an area of medical expertise and the current interest of psychologists and psychiatrists in 'spirituality' raises a real danger that they will assume unwarranted authority over the religious life of a patient.

While Gormally is right to criticize the way that 'health' (especially but not only 'reproductive health') is used to side-step moral considerations, and while his argument raises an important issue about the possibility of doctors assuming competence they do not possess in spiritual matters, his wish to confine health and well-being only to physical health is unpersuasive. It would effectively rule out the whole of psychiatry as a part of medicine. Furthermore, it should not be denied that human beings in general do have spiritual needs. Religion is so ubiquitous in different cultures and ages, even up to the present, that many have argued that there is a natural religious instinct in human beings. This is also supported by the Christian doctrine of creation and in different ways by other religions. There are also some aspects that different religions clearly share, and this is seen especially in the face of the existential threat of death (see for example CBCEW 2010).

Nevertheless, even a cursory knowledge of different faiths will show that as well as what is common there is also diversity between and indeed within every religious tradition. There is more than one religion and each religion is a complex cultural, social and intellectual reality. The danger of seeking to define a generic 'human spirituality' without relation to any specific religion is that this will be an abstraction and will do violence to the complexity of people's spiritual and religious lives. It may also become a kind of Esperanto – an artificial religion practised by no-one and created by healthcare professionals or authorities. Patients do indeed have spiritual needs and these will often be heightened by ill-health and the prospect of dependence or of death. However, to be adequately understood and addressed, these needs ultimately have to be interpreted in the context of the actual religious tradition through which patients understand themselves.

Religious Diversity and Non-Discrimination

The attempt of Koenig to demonstrate that religion is good for your health fails to do justice not only to the distinction some make between religion and spirituality, but more significantly, to the diversity of religion. Manifestly the effect of a religion on coping with ill-health will depend on the content of that religion and the particular way it has been assimilated by the patient (Kaldjian *et al.* 1998). Indeed it is arguable that a key way in which religion impacts upon medical practice is precisely that a doctor needs to take into account the diversity of religious belief and practice among patients, which may involve diverse needs or influence diverse responses.

Within the practice of medicine there is a movement, largely driven by ethical considerations, to empower patients to make their own healthcare decisions, and a concomitant movement away from 'the doctor knows best'. This movement to greater patient autonomy is not above criticism, but it has at least helped to clarify that, as is now widely acknowledged, best interest decisions cannot be reduced to considerations of clinical effectiveness. It is the patient who reaps the benefits, takes the risks and bears the burdens of medical intervention. It is the patient who has responsibility for his or her health and who integrates this responsibility with other responsibilities. It is the patient who must cope with ill-health, with dependency and with the approach of death. In making these decisions, integrating these responsibilities and facing these realities the patient is guided by a worldview which in many cases will be shaped in part by religion.

It is in the spirit of sensitivity to diversity of belief that the General Medical Council for the United Kingdom developed guidance on *Personal Beliefs and Medical Practice* (2008). This guidance acknowledges a diversity of beliefs among doctors and among patients and opposes all unfair discrimination on the basis of beliefs. Respecting patients' religious views is framed as a basic human right: 'You must respect patients' right to hold religious or other beliefs and should take those beliefs into account where they may be relevant to treatment options' (2008 para. 9). However, when the GMC comes to give examples of situations 'where patients' personal beliefs may affect care', the two examples given are: refusal of blood transfusion by Jehovah's Witnesses (paras. 10–11) and circumcision of male children for religious or cultural reasons (paras. 12–16). In the case of Jehovah's Witnesses the guidance makes clear their right to refuse treatment, but the emphasis falls on listening to the patient and not making assumptions. The guidance also makes physicians aware of the possibility of consulting with a hospital liaison committee established by the Watch Tower Society, where such exists. In the case of circumcision the guidance shows awareness of the opposition to the practice from anti-religious campaigners, but advises that the best interests of the child 'will include the child and/or his parents' cultural, religious or other beliefs and values.' (para 14). If both parents agree and if the doctor considers the procedure to be in the best interests of the child then it can be carried out. If a doctor objects then he must follow the general procedure for conscientious objection, including informing the parents of their right to a second opinion.

In both cases the GMC gives balanced and practical guidance, but it is immediately obvious that the GMC has taken examples where religious practice causes problems for the medical practitioner, and where the decision to refuse or to request treatment may seem unjustifiable on the basis of clinical considerations. It does not discuss examples where the religion of the patient may have a beneficial effect on the patient or where the role of the physician might include assessing spiritual need.

There are many possible ways in which religion may affect care and the focus on these examples effectively 'problematises' religion. This is also clear from the examples chosen of the way in which the personal beliefs of doctors may affect care. (Though the focus of the present chapter is on respecting the beliefs of patients, what the GMC guidance says about doctors helps clarify how religious beliefs of patients are being understood). In the case of doctors the guidance states that 'while we do not impose unnecessary restrictions on doctors, we expect them to be prepared to set aside their personal beliefs where this is necessary in order to provide care in line with the principles in Good Medical Practice' (2008 para. 8). The idea of 'setting aside' personal beliefs seems to assume that the moral and religious beliefs of the doctor should always be subordinated to the principles set out by the GMC. However, the guidance of the GMC gets its moral weight (as opposed to its legal sanction) only insofar as these embody true and adequate ethical principles. A doctor should not be expected to simply 'set aside' a personal belief if this concerns a commitment to an ethical principle. Here we encounter a general problem with the idea of setting limits to the toleration of conscientious objection, and how the community and the individual should respond to objections outside those limits.

The GMC guidance thus characterizes religion as subjective 'personal belief' that is potentially problematic for medical practice and seeks to negotiate the problem through the procedural justice of the patient's right to refuse treatment and the doctor's right to conscientiously object to giving treatment. While the importance of religious belief to people is acknowledged in general terms it is effectively invisible until it becomes a problem.

One should not be overcritical of the GMC for taking this approach for it is a repeated strand in the literature and no doubt also reflects the reasons that the guidance was requested. Nevertheless, the framing of the question in relation to 'problem cases' obscures the more general point that all medical practice involves decisions of best interest that are more complex than simple questions of clinical effectiveness, and all medical decisions take place within an ethical context. There is a rightful role here for procedural justice and for the ethics of managing ethical disagreement, but it would be naïve to think that the second order ethical principles of conflict resolution will be immune from ethical challenge. For example, the claim that a doctor has the right to object to providing treatment may itself be objected to by a patient. Similarly the refusal of a patient to cooperate in some matter, rather than *always* being respected, may lead to a threat of a wider withdrawal of care (unless, for example, the patient consents to be washed). It is not clear that such disputes can be resolved at an abstract level without some consensus as to what it is reasonable to object to. A better model for managing disagreements is set out in the GMC guidance on *Treatment and care towards the end of life*:

> If a patient asks you to provide nutrition or hydration by tube or drip, you should discuss the issues with the patient and explore the reasons for their request. You must reassess the benefits and burdens of providing the treatment requested, giving weight to the patient's wishes and values. When the benefits, burdens and risks are finely balanced, the patient's request will usually be the deciding factor. However, if after discussion you still consider that the treatment would not be clinically appropriate, you do not have to provide it. But you should explain your reasons to the patient and explain any other options that are available, including the option to seek a second opinion (2010 para. 117).

The clinical context here is a patient who can no longer swallow safely and who is requesting clinically assisted nutrition or hydration, but where the doctor does not think this would be effective. In the face of a request for treatment, rather than emphasizing that the patient has no right to demand treatment, the guidance draws attention to understanding the patient's reasons for the request. These reasons may include the religious or ethical significance the patient sees in, for example, the provision of food and fluids. The patient may believe that he or she has a religious duty to eat and may think of clinically assisted nutrition as fulfilling this duty. He or she might also feel the taking away of fluids as a kind of abandonment. Such beliefs and values will be an important element of the decision and the doctor should 'reassess' the decision in this better-informed moral context.

The doctor should explain the (limited) benefits of the intervention, and the risks, but it is the patient who takes the risks and the benefit may include a psychological benefit. Whereas some patients will feel a naso-gastric tube to be very burdensome and a medical intrusion, others may not regard it as especially burdensome and may regard it simply as a way to feed themselves. There may also be a difference here in how withholding or withdrawing is perceived. If the tube is already in place, a patient may not want this to be withdrawn. There is a dialogue here between moral and clinical considerations and the final decision requires both. This dialogue is a dialogue between experts, where each must be respectful of the views of the other. Clinical appropriateness is only part of the story in assessing overall best interests.

It is of course the case that a patient may doubt the particular clinical determination of the doctor, and may seek a second opinion. Analogously, where the view of the patient is explicitly influenced by religious considerations, there is a way in which this can be the subject of a 'second opinion' – by seeking the involvement of someone well-versed in the patient's religious tradition (who may be but need not be a hospital chaplain). The role of the religious advisor here is sometimes described as that of a translator – helping the doctor and patient understand each other better (see for example Orr and Genesen 1997). This was adverted to by the GMC in the specific case of Jehovah's Witnesses but it is a general consideration. Sometimes a religious figure can act as an interpreter or mediator.

To practice medicine ethically for the benefit of religious patients, religion should not be ignored or dismissed. While a doctor must not allow creed or religion to 'intervene' between the doctor and his or her duty to the patient, the patient's (and indeed the doctor's) religion may be relevant to establishing the nature of that duty. Religion informs the way the human good and thus the human needs of a patient are understood. Furthermore, religion is not only a personal or private matter but is also a public phenomenon that shapes communities, traditions, and patterns of reasoning, and in this way influences how patients understand and respond to the world, including their state of health.

When a patient is in a consultation with a doctor, should the doctor enquire about the patient's religious or spiritual beliefs? Clearly some patients wish doctors to inquire about this area (Ehman *et al.* 1999). Nevertheless, clearly not all do (Sloan *et al.* 2000). Doctors are in a position of power and patients are vulnerable in this respect as in other respects. This area requires sensitivity and is part of the wider requirement for doctors to understand the perspective of the patient. If religion influences the way patients make decisions and how they understand what is in their best interest, and if it is relevant to how patients respond to or cope with illness, then it is an area that doctors should be willing to explore. This is evident in the GMC guidance *Treatment and care towards the end of life* where doctors are told that discussion with patients who are dying *should* cover 'the patient's needs for religious, spiritual or other personal support' (GMC 2010 para 53(f))

The GMC thus requires doctors to be open to discussing religious and spiritual needs with patients, in this instance dying patients, but presumably these are not the only patients who have spiritual needs. This is not however to require that doctors share the same religious beliefs as their patients. In this context it is interesting to note new research from America which showed that psychiatrists, while their rate of religious practice was lower than other doctors, were much more aware of the importance of religion for patients, both as a potential problem and as a potential benefit. Hence, in comparison to other physicians, they were both more likely to think it appropriate to ask patients about spiritual matters (93% vs. 53%) and more likely to do so (87% vs. 49%). If a patient raises some spiritual or religious issue, psychiatrists will almost always take up the conversation (97%) whereas more than a quarter of other physicians will seek to change the subject (26%).[2]

It may well be that spiritual and religious concerns are more obviously relevant to psychiatry and to end of life care than to general medicine. Nevertheless, religion can have a very wide impact on decision making and on coping with illness. The physicians who are uncomfortable discussing this area, and who seek to change the subject, are failing to listen to their patients. Just as healthcare teams have become multi-disciplinary and frequently liaise with social care providers, so doctors should be aware of the patient's potential need for spiritual and/or religious support. This does not mean that the doctor is the primary provider of such support, this will come from chaplains, from relatives and carers, and, in some cases, from a faith community to which the patient belongs. Nevertheless, if a doctor is not the primary provider he or she should be aware of how religion may impact on healthcare decision making, on the patient's ability to cope with ill health, and on the needs a person may have in the face of ill health, isolation, disability, bereavement, or terminal illness.

Whatever is meant by responding to a religious or spiritual need, it cannot mean the physician denying his or her own beliefs (or lack of belief). Rather, what is required is a respect for the patient combined with an awareness of the existential challenge he or she faces, which may be understood by the patient in particular religious terms. If a doctor does not share that religious belief then it would be wrong to try to address this need directly in those terms. It would be and would feel inauthentic. Nevertheless, even without sharing the specific religious belief, there is much that the doctor can do, by listening without seeking to change the subject, and by being sensitive to the patient's wishes especially about small personal matters (CBCEW 2010 p. 17). It may be that someone from the same faith tradition can offer religious support in an explicit way. This is certainly something a doctor should be aware of and able to refer for (via chaplaincy services). Nevertheless, if this is not to make the patient feel to be an exercise in 'passing of the buck' then the doctor must also be willing to allow the spiritual conversation to take place, even while admitting that this is not his expertise.

It is perhaps easier to see how religion and spiritual issues arise in end of life care, and in psychiatry, but the vulnerability people feel in the face of death or mental disorder is present to a greater or lesser degree in all illness, and so these specialisms can offer some insights for the general physician. What is key is effective dialogue so as not to prejudge the shape that a shared understanding may take, but to listen to the other and to be ready to reassess one's own thinking in the light of what one learns from the process. It is through such a process that one learns what it means to respect the religious beliefs of the patient.

Chapter 10

Luck and Risk in Medicine

Nafsika Athanassoulis and Allison Ross

Luck and risk are both endemic in medicine – this is so because medical technology and practice are based upon knowledge of complex biological systems which is necessarily incomplete and leads to a level of unpredictability. The outcomes of both luck and risk can provoke strong reactions in patients, such as feelings of injustice, unfairness and being at the mercy of forces over which one has no control. Although, at first glance, both luck and risk may appear similar from the patient's perspective, it is worth distinguishing between the occurrences of the two phenomena in medical contexts. What both concepts have in common is that they are concerned with the nexus between decision-making agents on the one hand and the uncertain world in which they exist and act on the other. In this chapter we will try to outline the ways in which the two concepts differ.

Luck happens when events which have an impact upon a person's potential to pursue his interests are not under his control. The effect of these events can be positive or negative – producing good and bad luck respectively. So, for example, whether or not one is born with congenital blindness is something which impacts upon one's interests and life prospects and there is nothing one can do about it – it is a matter of luck.

Roughly speaking, while luck is something that happens to us, risk is something that we choose or that somebody else chooses on our behalf. Risk occurs when agents make choices and act in circumstances where they do not have full control over resultant events and consequently are uncertain what the actual outcome of their decisions and actions will be. Risk-takers have some idea about the possible outcomes of their choices but no way of being sure which outcome will be realized. Consider a patient who is going blind and who discovers that there is a form of surgery which has restored the sight of 50 per cent of those operated upon but has worsened it in 5 per cent of the cases. In addition past surgery has produced bad side effects in 12 per cent of the cases. She has no way of knowing whether she will be one of the successes and whether *she* will suffer side effects but she knows what is possible and what is improbable or likely. She must decide whether to take the risk in the pursuit of sight or not.

Risk-takers can be lucky or unlucky in the way things turn out but they understand this when they choose to risk and so are implicated in the causation of their resultant plight/status in a way that passive victims of luck are not. It is not always easy to disassociate risk and luck – in the above example we might say that that the woman who is going blind is unlucky to be going blind and to have to make a choice about whether or not to risk surgery. If she goes for surgery and things turn out badly we would still want to describe her as unlucky – but in this second instance of bad luck we would also say that she chose to risk its occurrence and therefore must bear some of the responsibility for her worsened situation. So where there is luck there is also likely to be risk and where there is risk, luck inevitably plays a part. Nevertheless, morally speaking, it is important to treat risk and luck differently – they give rise to different moral issues and consequently require different sorts of moral responses.

In this chapter, we will be considering and contrasting two cases, one involving luck and one involving risk, in order to compare the accounts of responsibility appropriate to each case.[1]

The diabetic patient: Deanne suffers from type 1 diabetes, a condition which needs to be carefully managed with insulin. Deanne is conscientious about following her blood testing and injecting regime, has made adjustments to her lifestyle to accommodate her condition, but still finds the injections painful and inconvenient. She has recently heard from her twin sister who suffers from the same condition, about the use of insulin pumps, which are painless, easy to use, discrete and overall sound far more appropriate for her requirements. However, her General Practitioner has advised her that the pumps are not available in her area. Deanne reflects on her bad luck; if only she lived in her sister's catchment area she would also be able to benefit from an insulin pump.

The prostate cancer patient: Thanos is a 60-year-old man who has just been diagnosed with prostate cancer. He has stage 2 cancer, which is good news in that the cancer has not spread to other sites, however, there are indications his cancer may grow swiftly, so a radical prostatectomy is indicated. On the other hand, Thanos suffers from asthma so has an increased risk of complications under general anaesthesia and he is very worried about the relatively small chance of side effects such as incontinence and erectile dysfunction as he has recently re-married.

What should these two patients do and how should they respond to the situations they find themselves in? Does Deanne have a cause for complaint for the lack of treatment? On what grounds should the decisions about Thanos' treatment be made? Does Deanne's perspective differ from Thanos'? To answer these questions and make sense of the different considerations which affect the two cases, we need to consider the differences between luck and risk.[2]

Luck

The notion of 'luck' is a particularly interesting one, but has received surprisingly little philosophical attention[3]. Occurrences due to luck happen by chance, without planning, control or design, perhaps unexpectedly and possibly outside the scope of individual responsibility, but at the same time they have a significant, either favourable or adverse, impact on the lives of those who experience them. The association of luck with lack of control seems to entail the claims that lucky outcomes are undeserved and that it is not fair to hold anyone responsible for them. We do not praise or blame people for being lucky, though we may congratulate or commiserate with them. Luck is also randomly distributed in unequal amounts and is consequently a source of undeserved differences in people's prospects – a result which can seem unfair. Consider the case of Deanne – if it is a matter of luck whether Deanne receives free treatment or not then this, on the face of it, seems unfair. Discrimination between her and others who live in a different place is undeserved and unjustifiable in any other way. A popular way of characterizing this sort of moral problem would be to say that Deanne is subject to a post-code lottery. In the UK there is strong public feeling against 'postcode lotteries' in treatment options presumably because they improperly subject patients to luck. It is worth noting that not all instances of luck would be considered unfair. If Deanne had come down with diabetes 10 years earlier than her sister when pumps did not exist and had to bear injections for 10 years then we would not think of Deanne as suffering unfairness. To properly consider why these initial judgements of fairness and unfairness occur and whether they are justified, we need to consider the notion of 'luck' in greater detail.

Many of the ways in which we employ the notion of 'luck' are entirely fabricated. We consider it bad luck to cross the path of a black cat, or good luck to follow a specific ritual before a significant event, or we worry that one's run of good luck cannot last forever. None of these beliefs relate to an actual phenomenon. Objects, rituals or past actions do not confer good luck as such, but rather reveal something about the psychological make-up of human beings (For more on this see Athanassoulis 2005 pp. 4–8). Even though we sometimes speak as if it is, luck is not a property; it cannot be conferred on an object or person, nor is it a phenomenon that can be consciously controlled.

Luck has two key elements – it concerns events and occurrences which affect individuals and it comes about because we lack control over these events and the ways in which they affect us. Lucky or unlucky occurrences are occurrences *for* someone whether beneficial or adverse. Many events take place outside of our control, but only the ones that affect us in a significant way can be described as lucky (Rescher 1995 pp. 19–20). Whether a particular event is indeed lucky or not will depend on the interests of those affected. Sometimes those affected have different and conflicting interests with the result that luck is differentially distributed. The sinking of the Spanish Armada by a storm in 1585 was a matter of bad luck for the Spanish and good luck for the English (*ibid. p. 20*). Where there are competing interests a single event can be an instance of good luck for some and bad luck for others. A medical example of similarly opposed interests differently served might be the case of a car accident victim who cannot be saved but can provide organs, the transplantation of which will save the lives of others.

Now let us turn to the 'accidental' quality of luck. Common sense associates 'luck' with events that are accidental or the product of chance. But the characteristic of chance or accident that we really seem to be referring to when we employ the concept of 'luck' is lack of control. Rescher defines luck as 'matter of our condition being affected, be it for good or ill, by developments that are neither intended nor foreseen, but lie substantially outside the domain of our control' (Rescher in Statman 1993 p. 146). We are inclined to think that accident/chance/lack of control over events must be a necessary condition of luck. This turns out not to be as obviously right as we might think. Consider Pritchard's objection to the relationship between luck and accident or chance. Pritchard argues that although the outcome of a lottery is a matter of luck, it need not necessarily be an accident that one wins. If one purposefully bought a ticket and chose one's numbers, their coming up on a Saturday night is not an accident in that one chose to buy the ticket and participate in the lottery with those numbers; one possible (although highly unlikely) outcome is a win for that person (Pritchard 2005 pp. 126–127). So the fact that an event is not accidental does not seem to entail that it is not also lucky. The appropriate response to Pritchard's challenge is to be more specific about what the lack of control inherent in luck involves. In fact, Rescher had already met this challenge head on – in his book he explains that the lack of control that opens the door to luck can arise in a variety of different ways – through the workings of chance, chaos, choice and ignorance (Rescher 1995 pp. 41–64).

Rescher identifies two kinds of chance. The first, which he calls 'strict' chance is the product of the fact that some events simply are under-determined and so need not have occurred exactly as they did. Randomness pervades some events including some of the most fundamental aspects of physics and there is no way to change this. In the face of such events prediction is not just impractical, it is categorically impossible. The second strand of 'chance' refers to the occurrence of anomalies – an event is said to be a product of chance when it is not what existing natural laws or norms would have led us to expect (Rescher 1995 pp. 43–44). Anomalies arise because of 'chaos', 'choice' and 'ignorance'. For Rescher's purposes chaos is defined as follows:

> A physical system is chaotic when its processes are so highly sensitive to conditions that very minute differences in an initial state can nevertheless engender very great differences in result, with miniscule local variations amplifying into substantial large-scale differences in the eventual outcomes (*ibid.* p. 45).

Examples of chaotic systems (in Rescher's sense of the word) might be living bodies, economies and institutions such as the NHS. Where there is chaos there is also luck because control of chaotic systems is impossible and also because absolutely accurate prediction of what they will do (while theoretically possible) is beyond us (*ibid.* p. 46). What Rescher is referring to, when he says that choice facilitates luck, is the way in which the free will of any of the agents involved in causally contributing to an event can potentially disrupt any expectations of how it will turn out. So where one is relying upon others to bring about an event there is an element of luck involved because nothing strictly necessitates that each of the others will play the requisite part.[4] Finally, ignorance about the nature of initial conditions, the workings of causation in a particular case or the likely results of a particular process inevitably means that much that is important to us is a product, at least in part, of luck. Because agents are ignorant of the causal mechanisms involved, from their perspective the outcome is as much beyond their control as it would have been if chance were involved. Ignorance undermines prediction and lack of prediction undermines any semblance of control (*ibid.* p. 50).

When we use the adjective 'accidental' to describe an event we mean that the event concerned is one where the persons affected by it are not in control of significant elements of the causal chain involved. For the reasons given above, being in control of significant elements of a causal chain is not a simple thing to achieve. As Dennett writes:

> Causation can be entirely inscrutable – utterly lost in a tangled web of coincidence – and still be causation . . . when we think of cases of causation we almost invariably think of cases where the relationships are laid bare, where the actuality or at least the practicality of control by an agent is manifest. Some cases of causation are called 'randomizing' processes precisely because of their uncontrollability (Dennett 1984 p. 60).

So causation is complex and unpredictable and we can have varying degrees of control over different processes. How does this help us respond to Pritchard's lottery example? The chain of causation that led to the individual lottery win is entirely inscrutable to the individual winner and beyond his power of influence, except in a very limited way (in that by buying the ticket he chooses to participate in the process that will lead to a winner, but this is an entirely different action from *choosing* to be that winner). So once he has the ticket – the rest, from his perspective, is a matter of luck. The notion of lack of control appropriate to luck is a very localized one and depends on the exact circumstances and the agent's relation to them.

Luck and Responsibility

Lucky (or unlucky) events are, by definition, events which impact upon agents but for which they are not responsible.[5] So for example Deanne is not responsible for the fact she does not have access to insulin pumps. Lack of responsibility for good or ill luck holds even though the agents concerned may have had some small power to influence events. What matters is whether one has control over the significant determinants of an event. Deanne has some control over her situation – she could have chosen to locate herself in the same area as her sister. However, in this case we take it that the significant determinants of the situation regarding the distribution of insulin pumps are the National Health policy makers. These bodies occupy a social role with which comes a clearly defined sphere of responsibility – one that includes the differential distribution of insulin pumps. Because this is the way our society is organized, the distribution of pumps falls outside Deanne's sphere of responsibility. Spheres of responsibility are determined by normative considerations – they follow from duties that arise because of the way society is organized or because of the existence of other stake-holders, etc. This provides us with an important insight into the 'significant influence over causation' to which we referred above. It tells us that significance is determined in part by normative considerations. This is why there is such a strong link between luck and non-responsibility – the one entails the other. That is also why, very often, in order to work out whether an event is lucky we first consider whether we think the beneficiary is responsible for it. The notions of 'culpability' and 'negligence' all rely on how one judges the agent's responsibility for accidental events and such judgements can vary according to normative situations.

Nobody is responsible for their good or bad luck. However, the presence of luck in our daily lives is something we are conscious of and which we have a responsibility to respond sensibly to. In particular we can have a responsibility to others to do everything in our power to ensure that our actions do not introduce the prospect of bad luck into their lives where this was avoidable. It is one thing to be affected by luck that is the result of natural process and another to be affected by luck that is created by human carelessness or human artifice.

Part of taking up a responsible attitude to luck involves seeking to gain as much control as possible over events (especially those which affect others) in a way that limits the exposure of ourselves and those in our care to luck. Diminishing the role of luck by avoiding negligence and ignorance (of what could be reasonably known) is also important. A doctor who neglects to find out whether a patient is diabetic before prescribing other medication illegitimately introduces more vulnerability to luck into that patient's life. Similarly a GP who does not keep up to date on the latest medical technologies may leave a patient languishing in the realm of luck when this is unnecessary.

A second way in which we can adopt a responsible attitude to luck involves structuring our social world in ways that make individual people or groups more or less subject to luck. The extent to which luck ought to be allowed to affect groups of people is quite controversial – it is the subject matter of distributive justice. Libertarians hold that we have no responsibility to limit or ameliorate the effects of luck (Nozick 1974 p. 225 ff.). Egalitarians, on the other hand, tend to hold that it is the responsibility of the powerful to ensure that the unlucky are not excessively disadvantaged by their ill-luck (Cohen 1989 pp. 907–932). These sorts of debate have found expression in medical ethics in the debate about post-code lotteries among other things.[6]

Earlier we observed that, intuitively, there seemed to be something unfair about Deane's ill-luck and that of other victims of post-code lotteries. That intuition can be explained now by appeal to the egalitarian assumptions that under write it. Those who think Deanne has been treated unfairly think so because they hold that the National Health Service (NHS) has a duty to distribute its resources in accordance with the immediate health needs of individuals, regardless of non-health criteria such as geography. On such a view the NHS' sphere of responsibility is structured by an egalitarian requirement of justice. Those who think that Deanne's ill-luck is not unfair think of the sphere of responsibility of the NHS as being structured by the normative requirement to maximize the tailoring of local services to local needs. They see the only justice requirement structuring the responsibility of the NHS to be one of procedural fairness in which policies are transparent and consistently applied.[7] Here there is some dispute over the type of responsibility the NHS has and disagreement over what counts as adopting a responsible attitude to luck.

A third way in which we can be responsible in the face of a future partly determined by luck is to exercise discipline in choice. Facing up to the prospect of luck and making decisions, knowing that luck will play a part in how things turn out is rational risk-taking. The nature of rational risk-taking is complex and raises moral issues peculiar to itself. We consider risk-taking and its implications for responsibility in the following section.

Risk

Risk as a concept has a much stronger connection to agency and responsibility than luck. While there is a valid distinction between risks we face, e.g. natural disasters, and risks we take, e.g. choosing to build in a flood plain (Rescher 1983 pp. 5–6), the interesting aspects of risk are those which involve choice and the risks we choose to take. The term risk is, in its primary sense, a verb rather than the description of a phenomenon. 'Risk' describes a decision to pursue a course of action that exposes one to uncertain outcomes in the hopes of either achieving good results or avoiding bad ones. Crucially while there is an element of deliberation about one's decision to become involved in risk-taking, and therefore it is appropriate to judge the outcomes of such deliberation as reasonable or not, the results of risk will always be subject to uncertainty. Risk then involves an ineliminable tension between the responsibility inherent in the decision making to participate in risk and the lack of control (or total control) over the uncertain outcomes.

Unlike luck, risk is not something that happens to us, but something that we choose to become involved in. We can deliberate as to options and may be held responsible for the reasonableness of our decision to participate in the risk (For more on this see Ross and Athanassoulis 2011). The outcome of risk is not the most significant part of the evaluation of the agent's behaviour, as the decision to undertake the risk may in itself display poor judgement regardless of the outcome. Consider, for example, a doctor who decides to take the risk of getting drunk with a visiting friend when he is on-call and has every reason to expect that he may well have a busy night looking after emergency patients. Should it turn out that, due to a stroke of luck, he is not called out to treat anyone, we would not want to conclude that he was therefore justified in taking the risk in the first place. It is his decision to risk the life of the patients under his care for a reason as frivolous as personal enjoyment of the effects of alcohol, that we should hold him responsible for and that which displays his faults of character, i.e. his callousness as to the welfare of others and his predominantly self-interested attitude in situations where he has a duty of care to others (For more on this see Athanassoulis and Ross, forthcoming).

Of course, making assessments about the reasonableness of one's decisions with respect to risk will be an extremely complicated process, subject to many different factors, contexts, situational particulars, etc. and requiring both maturity and delicacy of judgement (For more on this see Ross and Athanassoulis, forthcoming). Good risk-taking or risk-avoidance requires good character which, in turn, involves wisdom and well-regulated feelings and desires. These are the things that the drunk doctor lacks and it is for their absence, which manifests as carelessness and callousness, that we blame him.

For the purposes of our discussion, what matters is the difference in the way in which luck and risk relate to responsibility. The notion of lack of control, inherent in our definition of luck, suggests that judgements of responsibility are not appropriate for those who are subject to luck. However, this is not the case for decisions involving risk, for although the outcomes of risk are uncertain, we can have knowledge of the possibilities, the probabilities and the factors which affect risk. In addition, risk is something we choose knowingly – in full understanding that the outcome of our choice is uncertain. Therefore when one risks one has reasons for doing so which either validate or invalidate one's decision to participate in the risk.

Thanos is unlucky because he is faced with a difficult choice – he must do one of two things both of which involve risks. To have the operation would be to risk the occurrence of a) potentially serious complications of anaesthesia and b) distressing post-operative side-effects which may impact substantially upon his quality of life. The benefit of taking risk A is that his cancer will be eliminated from his body and the chances of recurrence (after radiotherapy) would be very small indeed. Not to remove the tumour (risk B) would expose Thanos to the risk that the cancer would spread and bring about his premature death within about 5–10 years. The advantage of not operating would be that he would avoid the perils of anaesthesia and retain his quality of life and the prospect of holding on to his new wife. How ought a decision to be made concerning whether the operation should take place? In this case we have a combination of pure bad luck and the potential to exacerbate or ameliorate the bad situation created by luck by taking a risk. Nobody can be blamed for the fact that Thanos finds himself in this situation. However, somebody may well be blame-worthy if his situation is worsened as a result of choices made for inadequate or bad reasons.

We noted above that individual agents can be held responsible for their risk-involving choices. How do we go about assigning responsibility and where appropriate moral praise and blame? Some moral philosophers might suggest that Thanos ought (morally) to choose the option with the best chances of a good outcome. However this is a problematic strategy partly because in this case it is debateable what the best outcome is. The oncologist may think that it is freedom from cancer and from the constant threat of death. Thanos, on the other hand, might value the guarantee of up to 5 years of life in which he will be able to do what he wants to do more. In addition, even if we could agree that operation had the greatest probability of producing the best outcome the crude consequentialist strategy would still be problematic for similar reasons to the doctor case above.

We think a better strategy for attributing responsibility for risk-taking involves consideration of the detailed reasons for which risk decisions are made. Thanos has been presented with a particularly difficult choice – he does not have the choice not to risk because even 'doing nothing' involves taking risks. There are any number of reasons he might go for one or other of the options. He might, for example, be very afraid of anaesthesia or distrustful of surgeons having lost a loved one 'under the knife'. These feelings could be proportionate and reasonable or disproportionate and unreasonable depending upon the details of his actual situation. Alternatively he may have researched the potential for asthmatic complications under anaesthetic and have discovered a study which suggests the probabilities of such complications are higher than the standard estimates. Once again many variables would be involved in determining how reasonable it is to place weight on this study in the course of his decision. A third alternative might be that that he values his life because it offers him the opportunity to enjoy his new marriage – not being impotent may be central to his own conception of the sort of husband he wants to be. For generous reasons he may not wish his new wife to suffer many years with an increasingly miserable husband and prefer the option of a few years of what he sees as a good quality life together. A good quality decision will be one in which his feelings, beliefs and desires are balanced and all cohere in favour of the same course of action.

All this may sound rather vague and unsatisfactory if our concern is what is the best decision for Thanos to make. However this may be a problem with the subject matter itself. The question of the justification of Thanos's decision cannot be answered without knowing all these myriad of details and being able to assess all the particulars which make this decision unique as made by this distinct individual. It is our view that no 'simple decision procedure' can provide simple answers concerning the rightness or wrongness of a choice to risk (Athanassoulis and Ross 2010). The difficulty of assessing the justifiability of the decision should not detract from the fact, though, that the decision can be justified or unjustified and that this will be so irrespective of the outcome of the decision. Had Thanos made an entirely flippant, uneducated and not particularly reflective decision to risk, but been lucky enough not to suffer any negative consequences, we would still hold him responsible for the quality of his decision. Matters which seriously affect one's health and have repercussions for one's loved ones and for the medical professionals involved in one's care, require a certain amount of careful consideration and dedicated attention. Thanos could be held responsible for being flippant and fickle, regardless of whether he ever suffered the consequences of his flippancy.

Risk is intrinsic to medicine: patients seek out medical attention to avert the risk of suffering and death and there are few responses in the arsenal of medical practitioners that are entirely risk-free. Moral questions arise concerning who the risk-choosers ought to be and what choices to risk (or not) are good quality choices. Answering the first type of question invokes considerations of autonomy, the permissibility of paternalism, etc. which we cannot discuss here. Answering the second sort of question requires special focus upon the practical rationality of one particular chooser. At the core of the ethics of risk, then, lies a decision. It is the quality of that decision, the coherence of the moral psychology manifested in making it, that determines whether the risk-taking, in any particular case, is morally acceptable. The quality of such practical decision-making is difficult but not impossible to assess. Among the considerations that will need to be taken into account are context or circumstances, details about persons whose decision it is (their views, their volitions, the role occupied when taking the decision, etc.) as well as details about the persons who will be affected by it – the decision to risk. Responsibility for risk is responsibility for the process which generated the choice – where that process is based upon incomplete grasp of the situation and persons affected or unduly influenced by prejudice, or more than reasonable fear or self-interest, or some such motive then we can blame the risk-chooser for taking the risk when they ought not to have or for failing to risk when they ought to have done so.

Conclusion

So luck is a ubiquitous phenomenon which means that the future well-being of people is uncertain. Risk is a response to the need to act in the context of uncertainty. Luck is not anyone's fault but there are ways of influencing the degree to which persons are subject to luck at both the policy and the personal level. There is probably a justice imperative to seek to balance out the effects of luck to prevent inequality. Where this is so the responsibility will fall to those involved in policy making. There is a care imperative for medical practitioners to ensure that luck is not at play where this is avoidable i.e. to insure that they are well-informed and well-skilled in their practice. However, on the whole being the victim of luck, while unjust and often devastating is not praise or blame-worthy. By contrast risk is actively chosen and therefore the subject of full moral evaluation. Different philosophers have different ideas about how such moral evaluation should take place. We have pursued a virtue ethics approach to the evaluation of risk which suggests that the relevant evaluations are evaluations of character and will be highly context-sensitive.

This different analysis of luck and risk accounts for our different perspectives towards the two cases we considered. Deanne is at the mercy of forces that she has absolutely no control over and outcomes she has no responsibility for. A sense of frustration, impotence and unfairness is appropriate, especially under situations where luck has been allowed unlimited influence with no attempt to mitigate its unjust results. Thanos is more in control of his destiny and although also potentially subject to negative outcomes, he can be held responsible for the reasonableness of the decisions that he makes with respect to risk.

Chapter 11

The Lay Patient and Genetic Illness

Ruth Stirton[1]

'You Have the BRCA Predisposition to Breast Cancer'

Eight words that strike fear into the person hearing them. Developments in genetic testing means that more women can expect to hear this in the future. Worryingly, most of us will not be adequately prepared for this sort of news.

This chapter explores philosophical literature covering the rights and duties surrounding knowledge, the specialness of genetic information, and the potential for discrimination arising from its use. I suggest that this literature minimizes, and to some extent ignores, the patient at the centre of the experience of genetic illness and genetic testing. I argue that the phenomenological philosophy of Husserl, Heidegger and Merleau-Ponty offers an alternative to the more usual analytical moral philosophical approach. Specifically, its value comes from its focus on the subjective lived experience and perceptions of the patient at the centre of the question. Having a deeper understanding of the patient's experiences will give a more robust grounding from which moral philosophers can develop better normative principles. I consider some of the more recent uses of phenomenology in understanding health and illness, and illustrate (briefly) how more of this work could be carried out.

Duties to know and rights not to know

The question of how much or how little information a person should be required to know about their genetic makeup has occupied philosophers for a long time. Broadly speaking, there are two schools of thought. One school argues that individuals are under a duty to find out as much as they can about their genetic makeup. This duty could mean that it is rational to know everything about yourself, and you should seek out information, or more worryingly, that your duty to know entails a duty on others to tell you, and perhaps to collect information about you with the express purpose of telling you. The first does leave room for some individual autonomy since it might be rational in some situations for a person to choose not to know, whereas the second could have come straight from the dystopia in George Orwell's *Nineteen Eighty-Four*. The other school argues that the individual has a right not to know information about themselves. This could be a negative right imposing a duty on others not to impose information on the individual, or a substantive right in which the individual must have real and admirable reasons for their decision not to know. Rosamond Rhodes (1998 p.18), a Kantian proponent of the duty to know, argues that people can only make fully autonomous decisions about how to live their lives if they are in possession of the fullest possible knowledge about themselves. Therefore, there can be no right not to know. Rhodes understands 'right' to mean the existence of a moral freedom to decide on the matter. She argues that there can be no moral freedom in this situation; rather, one is under an 'obligation to pursue genetic knowledge' (Rhodes 1998 p. 17). It is far from clear how she expects this duty to be enforced. Despite considerable challenge (Takala 1999; Takala and Häyry 2000), Rhodes (2000) stands by this view. One conceptual difficulty with her argument is her distinctions between types of decisions. Rhodes does not doubt that decisions about treatment are decisions which can be made autonomously: in fact, her duty to know is premised on protecting the patient's ability to make maximally autonomous treatment decisions. However, she denies that any decision to be made prior to a treatment decision is one that can be made autonomously. She seems to deny that these are decisions at all. The patient simply does as they are told by their healthcare provider. If we think about what is involved in undergoing predictive genetic testing in the NHS – starting with a GP appointment, then a referral to a genetics clinic, then genetic counselling before the test – there seems to be no question that the decision whether to undergo testing is at least as significant as a treatment decision. If a testing decision is a decision that can be made autonomously, then the decision maker must have a real opportunity to make a choice. There cannot be a requirement to decide in a particular way. Rhodes' duty to know dictates to patients the course of action they must follow in all situations prior to medical treatment decisions. There is no scope for individual decision-making, because the correct decision has already been made. Even if the arguments for it are grounded in a conception of autonomy, this seems to be so antithetical to what is meant by autonomous decision-making, that it is almost nonsensical to argue for this duty.

Tuija Takala (1999) and Juha Räikkä's (1998) alternate view, is that a person has a right not to know about their genetic risk, which includes a right not to undergo predictive genetic testing. They ground their rights in Mill's harm principle – persons are free to make their own decisions and act in their chosen manner, however apparently irrational, except insofar as those actions or decisions do not harm others (Räikkä 1998 p. 59; Takala and Häyry 2000 p. 108). If the decision not to find out this information will not harm others, then the individual is free to choose not to know. This necessarily imports the definitional difficulties associated with the concept of harm in Mill's principle. When considering reproductive decisions, it is not clear if it is possible to harm the unborn, whether this refers to an identifiable foetus or unidentifiable future generations (Takala 1999 p. 290). Neither is it clear if a decision not to have a predictive genetic test could harm existing persons, e.g. by failing to prepare friends and relatives or to provide for dependants. If there is no way of harming another person, then there is no conceptual way to restrict the decisions that people can make.[2] This makes it very difficult to talk about a right (not) to know.

For both these schools, the morally significant issue is whether a person has decided to have a test or not. To my mind, this places the focus too far in the future. If we are concerned about individual autonomy, whether Millian or Kantian, then the decision itself is most important. The right (not) to know hints at this, but I would argue that it is important for the promotion of individual autonomy that there is a right to make your own decision, in the manner of your choosing. I would argue that the individual is best placed to know who and what is important to them when making decisions about genetic testing or other healthcare options. Giving proper thought to who and what is important allows the individual to make the decision which takes into account the interests of those she considers to be important and to affect her choices. For example, if a person's concern is about passing on a condition to the next generation, but she has already decided not to have children, then it would be legitimate to decide not to know. Likewise, if she already has children, there is nothing she can do to change whether she has passed the condition on, so it might be legitimate to decide not to have a test, rather to talk to the children about it when they are able to understand. The important thing is recognising that these are legitimate options. The best way to do that is to protect the individual's ability to make the decision themselves, rather than advocating an approach which entails someone else making a decision for them.

The X factor?

Another question occupying academic commentators is about the nature of genetic information. There is a general intuition that genetic information is special in some way, and that this unknown X factor provides regulators with a good reason for considering genetic information differently from other personal information. Much of this work argues that our DNA provides a blueprint for our development: a 'future diary' (Annas 1999 p. 11). This oracle is so important to the way we choose to live our lives that it should be subject to special levels of protection (Richards 2001). This argument appeals to our general obsession with knowing the future – illustrated by our use of fortune tellers and horoscopes. If our DNA could accurately predict the future, then this might be a good reason for stringent regulation of its use. The biological reality is that DNA is dependent on other developmental processes, and is affected by other biological functions and environmental factors. The way DNA is discussed in the media perpetuates the view that it is the only factor that is relevant to our futures. Discussions of DNA in terms of communication technology analogies emphasizes the myth that our genome is like a CD holding the secrets of our humanity. The notion of the 'future diary' may have obfuscated our view of the nature of information about our genetic makeup.

A second way in which it is argued that genetic information is different from other types of health information is its familial nature. Information about my genetic makeup can also reveal something about my relatives' genetic makeups. I might, perhaps unwittingly, come to know something about my parents, children or siblings as a result of my own test information. Loane Skene argues that the model which sees information about genetics as family-owned information rather than individual information might eventually be more protective of the individual's rights (Skene 1998 p. 40). This communitarian model, where the information belongs to the family community, provides that individuals do not have full control over what happens to the information. Rather, healthcare professionals have a duty to share it with the family members. Skene argues that this model takes better account of the reality of treating families with genetic conditions, and that it is better focused on health promotion than the traditional individualistic model (Skene 1998 p. 34). Specifically, it makes tissue and information more readily available to other family members. Dean Bell and Belinda Bennett (2001) argue that this communitarian model goes too far. Merely having a genetic affiliation with another person is not a sufficiently strong conception of family to require a change in the ethical and legal codes that govern the disclosure of this information (Bell and Bennett 2001 p. 132). As Jan Trost (1990) shows, there are many possible understandings of the concept of family, much wider than just those with whom we share our genes. If we take the genetic family as the standard notion of family, then children and parents have a right to be involved in the use of information, but spouses and stepchildren do not. If the relevant notion of family is those who live together, then this would exclude adult children who have left home, or grandparents, for example. If we are going to follow the route that says information is familial, not just individual, we need a clear idea of who the relevant family members are.

Bell and Bennett (2001) argue further that protection of family members does not require a move away from an individualistic model, since individuals do not make decisions merely on the basis of abstractions. Individual autonomy should be seen in the context of the relationships of which the individual is part (Bell and Bennett 2001 p. 158). Since this is the case, the individual is best placed to know which relationships are important to the decision they are making, and can be trusted to take account of those interests in the decision-making process.[3]

While this is one argument for the distinctiveness of genetic information, this is not the only health information that provides information about someone else. As Michael Green and Jeffrey Botkin (2003 p. 572) argue, other tests can have implications for, or tell us something about other people. Blood tests for infectious diseases may indicate that those who have been in close contact with us may also be at risk, and positive results for sexually transmitted diseases will also tell us something about the health of our sexual partners. It is not immediately clear whether knowing your sister's risk of breast cancer is more or less devastating for you or her, than knowing your partner's risk of having HIV. If one type of test is to be treated differently at a regulatory level, then there should be a good reason for the difference.[4]

These two areas are two of the main contenders for the X factor. The discussion is far from closed. Philosophers are rarely comfortable accepting intuition as a justification for a view that something is important. There is considerable work still to be done. It may be that we are still too near to the beginning of genetic discovery and understanding to be able to clearly see genetics as anything other than something shrouded in mystery. Once further research has helped to expel that mystery, and has elucidated and communicated the links between genetic predispositions, biology and environment, the mystical X factor may turn out to be something much more pedestrian. Societies in the distant future may well wonder what all the fuss was about.

Genetic discrimination

There is no universally accepted definition of the concept of genetic discrimination; rather there is almost universal disagreement about the nature of the concept.[5] While the precise terms are proving difficult to pin down, the core of the issue is that people should not be denied access to something they would ordinarily have been entitled to, on the basis of information about their genetics. The literature identifies three main areas where discrimination could arise: employment, provision of healthcare, and access to goods and services such as insurance.

The problem is of particular concern in states where healthcare is not fully socialized, since access is governed by a person's insurance cover. In many situations, health insurance is an employment benefit paid for by the employer. Predictive genetic information about employees or potential employees could significantly increase the cost of health insurance, and thus the cost to the employer of the insurance premium. A significant concern was that employers would use genetic information as a reason to terminate the contracts held by existing employees or for not employing job applicants (Miller 2000). On the one hand it seems unjust to deny someone employment because of something unrelated to their ability to do the job. Equally, a small organization could be placed under significant financial pressure by the insurance premiums payable for someone with a known genetic predisposition. It is easy to see that companies might succumb to this reasoning, especially in a difficult economic climate. The US has enacted the Genetic Information Nondiscrimination Act 2008, which prohibits discrimination in employment, and in the provision of health insurance on the basis of genetic information.[6] It will take some time to see the effects of this new Act, but the first claim has already been widely publicized.[7] In early 2010, Pamela Fink made a claim against her employer MXenergy. She claims that declaring her positive BRCA test and a short absence from work for risk-reducing surgery caused her employment to be terminated. Prior to this she was an exemplary employee. On her return she received very negative reviews despite continuing to work in the same way. As yet, the case remains undecided.

The issue for the UK is the provision of goods and services, specifically, life insurance (Low *et al.* 1998).[8] For many, some life cover is essential to buying a house and is certainly a wise investment when considering starting a family. Premiums are currently assessed on the basis of family and individual medical histories, and there is a voluntary moratorium in place in which the insurance industry has agreed not to ask for predictive genetic test information (Department of Health 2005).[9] The concern is that if insurance companies are allowed to ask applicants to disclose predictive genetic test information, then people will choose not to have medically indicated tests, and that those who do disclose this information will be denied insurance cover (Ashcroft 2007; Holm 2007). The difficulty in the UK is knowing whether insurance discrimination is a serious problem. Low *et al.*'s (1998) study undertaken prior to the moratorium showed some preliminary empirical evidence that genetic discrimination was occurring in a non-systematic way in the UK life insurance market. It is unclear whether the problem would have developed further or disappeared without the moratorium or whether discrimination would have become more systematic if the moratorium was allowed to expire. The difficulty faced in the UK is that we need to know much more about what the problem of genetic discrimination involves before it will be possible to address it. There is nothing comparable to Low *et al.*'s (1998) work which could tell us what is happening now. Without a clear picture of the current position or what people are concerned about when they talk about genetic discrimination, there is no hope of settling on a coherent national policy. Much more work is needed before this could be achievable.

The Lay Patient and their Genetic Illness

This book focuses on the real interactions between patients and doctors. As should be evident, the philosophical literature on this area takes an objective standpoint, discussing the problem of genetic illness in an abstract manner, divorced from the experiences of the patients at its centre. This is the same challenge as that made by Edmund Husserl in the early twentieth century. He argued that philosophers were too concerned with abstract problems, and that subjectivity and the 'concrete living experience' (Moran 2000 p. xiii) had at least as much to offer to philosophical endeavours. Although the work on the right not to know and the right to decide offers some recognition of the patient, much of the rest starts at a stage far removed from the patient. The right to choose is most relevant to patients whose rights are being threatened, and the discrimination discussion becomes relevant once a patient is at risk of discrimination. For the patient sitting in the clinic waiting for test results, these questions are too distant from the experience and may obfuscate the problems they face, rather than help to clarify their position. If you are unable to see through the issues to make a decision, then knowing that you have a right to protect that decision is not going to help clear your mind.

If we refocus on the patient, and consider the questions that might help us to help her to deal with her genetic illness, we could start with the question of 'what does the word "genetic" mean to the patient?' Gaining a real understanding of what the lay patient hears when the word 'genetic' is uttered will identify a path to follow. There is a paucity of work on this question. Martin Richards and Maggie Ponder found some evidence that the general public had a poor understanding of genetics and genetic illness. Lay people tended to lack an understanding of fundamental biological realities, such as the difference between genotype and phenotype (Richards and Ponder 1996 p. 1033). Further work carried out by Susan Cox and William McKellin (1999) in Huntington's Disease families showed that those who live with their genetic risk in the background see it as an inescapable part of their family but do not consider the objective complexities of the position they are in, such as the specific financial and reproductive implications of their condition. They focus on the risk that individuals face from being a member of the family, rather than the concept of genetics itself. If we consider Evelyn Parsons and Paul Atkinson's (1992) work in which they talked to women at risk of passing on Duchenne Muscular Dystrophy, it becomes apparent that the lay patient shies away from the scientific details surrounding the condition. Instead they reconceptualized their understanding of the problem into 'meaningful everyday statements' (Parsons and Atkinson 1992 p. 446) about reproductive options. This highlights issues about the need for certainty, and the existential difficulty of living in a state of uncertainty. Mairi Levitt (2003) indicates the problem with this work, arguing that methodological choices are made for reasons which may not be wholly positive. Written questionnaires are used when the purpose is to show that the public have a poor understanding, and need education. Interviews are used when there is an interest in what the patient thinks. The research methodology may indicate significant bias towards particular conclusions. Furthermore, the results are highly context-linked, and do not shed much light on the experiences of the individual genetics patient that we are focusing on. If philosophers are to engage with the experiences and difficulties of patients, then more work needs to be done to explore what their genetic risk means to them and how they cope with discovering a genetic predisposition to a serious illness.

A new research agenda?

Phenomenology offers us the ability to engage with the subjective experiences of patients suffering from genetic illness. It is a radical philosophical methodology which offers a serious challenge to the third-person approach espoused in the more traditional philosophical schools (Moran 2000 p. xiv). It allows us to explore the essence of the individual's experience, and to draw conclusions about the nature of their existence. Rather than taking the external position favoured by analytical moral philosophers, phenomenology moves the philosopher to the inside, using the individual's perceptions and experiences to form theories about what is happening. Husserl's method of phenomenological philosophy requires the philosopher to bracket or suspend any theories or views they already hold, and start their investigations 'in absolute poverty, with an absolute lack of knowledge' (Husserl, *Cartesian Meditations* 1, 2 Hua I 44).

The relationship between the patient and their healthcare provider is a paradigmatic example of objectivity masking the real experiences of individuals. This is especially so when one considers the organizational complexity of modern healthcare provision. It is unsurprising that the patient's perspective often gets lost. In *Limits to Medicine,* Ivan Illich presents an image of modern medicine as a self-constituting and self-regulating social system, which constructs individual states and internal conditions as illness. The health care system in this way abstracts from the individual perspective, reconstructing the patient's complaint in abstract medical terms, *medicalizing* conditions that would otherwise be interpreted as part of the life world. In his preface to the 1995 edition of *Limits to Medicine,* Illich confesses his remorse about the impact of his account of healthcare:

> I was unaware that by construing health in this self-referentially cybernetic fashion, I unwittingly prepared the ground for a worldview in which the suffering person would get even further out of touch with the flesh. I neglected the transformation of the experience of body and soul when well-being comes to be expressed by a term that implies functions, feedbacks and their regulation (Illich 2002 p. iii).

Illich was concerned about the machinery of healthcare provision dehumanizing patients, but the concern applies to those considering the philosophy of healthcare provision: if the patients are dehumanized or even ignored, then how can we construct an adequate normative account of patients' experience of the health care system?

It should be apparent that phenomenology has something to offer which could enrich philosophical work. Despite this, there is a dearth of philosophical research using the phenomenological method. A particularly good example is Havi Carel's book *Illness: The Cry of the Flesh* (2008), in which she uses Maurice Merleau-Ponty's embodied personhood concept as a starting point for understanding her experiences as a sufferer of lymphanfioleiomyomatosis, an incurable lung disease which significantly reduces life expectancy. Carel starts by arguing that the problem with illness is that it disrupts the harmony between the objective biological body and the lived experience of the body. In a healthy person, these two should be seamlessly aligned (*ibid.* p. 26). This disharmony focuses the patient's attention on the malfunctioning body. In health, the body exists in the background and does not intrude into the person's considerations: it can be relied on to perform. Illness changes the biological body, which forces a change to the lived experience of the body. She argues that this change is fundamental to our existence as a person: it 'strikes at the heart of subjectivity' (*ibid.* p. 29). The next theme she considers is the social experience of illness, focusing on interactions with doctors and the rest of society. In the first, the issue is the different languages spoken by doctors and patients. Doctors are impersonal and objective, where patients are personal and subjective (*ibid.* p. 39). It is possible that this difference is grounded in the division between the objective and subjective bodies, with doctors focusing on the objective biological body, and the patients focusing on the subjective lived body. It raises questions about which language is more important, and a chronically ill patient could be forgiven for thinking that her treatment experiences would be better if she could speak the language favoured by her healthcare provider. The changes to the body also have negative effects on social perception. Intimate details of your life are on show for all to see (*ibid.* p. 58). It is interesting to see how others deal with this. It could either become common property which is used by strangers to define us, or be conspicuously absent from relationships with others. It is not clear which is worse. The final theme which emerges throughout Carel's work is the question of health within illness or whether a person can be ill and happy. This is particularly important for the chronically ill patient where illness is a persistent part of life. Carel argues that creative responses and adaptability are fundamental to a chronic patient's experience of happiness (*ibid.* p. 81). This adaptation or coping with the challenges means that the patient reframes the narrative of their life to take account of the illness. It is at least arguable that a shortened life expectancy could in some ways help a patient who is forced to see their life as finite, and who may therefore be able to commit themselves to live in the present. It is possible that a shortened life lived in the now is preferable to a longer life in which the person defers important experiences to their future.

A phenomenological exploration of experiencing genetic illness

To illustrate the type of work that I think needs to be done to further flesh out this area, I have analyzed internet forum posts related to genetic illnesses and genetic testing. At this stage, I offer no more than an indication of the sort of phenomenological research that could form the basis of a future research agenda.

I focused on seventeen forum threads from two well-known UK-based parenting support websites. I chose threads that specifically focused on genetics questions. Each thread had the same basic structure. A website user, who may choose to post anonymously or using their pseudonymous screen name, posts a question or a story and invites replies from other website users. In order to reply to a thread, you have to register and log in to the website, but there is no such restriction on reading the posts. Everything written is fully available to the public. One of the websites has 'health visitors' and 'parent supporters' who offer something akin to professional advice to the original poster throughout some of the discussion threads. The rest of those posting in response to questions occasionally provide some details indicating a professional understanding of the issues involved, but are not engaging in a professional capacity. The general impression of the data is that this is a group of people who have had some similar experiences, and reply through a feeling of solidarity with those who raise questions.

The lived experience of genetic illness

Most of the forum posts considered were posted by individuals who had recently discovered their genetic risk. They were often 'upset and frightened' or in 'shock' over the news they had received. This anxiety was often grounded in the uncertainty of their situation, the feeling that they could not rely on their bodies to support them: 'you have momentarily lost that certainty about your life'. Once that thought was raised, it led people to think more deeply about the general lack of certainty in human existence. The problem with this specific uncertainty is not that it is something new or special, rather that it brings the uncertainty of life to the foreground, and particularly highlights the limits of mortality: 'I've always been scared of dying anyway and this has reawoken those fears'. The uncertainty, coupled with the pressure to make the right decision about whether to have a test or not, creates a feeling of isolation from and difference to other people: 'I feel so isolated from the rest of the world knowing that their lives will progress normally while mine probably won't'. It is this isolation or feeling of disconnectedness that encourages them to seek contact with other people. The support of others can be a very positive experience: 'I personally would like to thank everyone on this forum who have contributed; it makes me feel I am not alone in all this'. This need to connect flows both ways, there are many contributions from people who have already experienced similar problems whose main reason for contributing is that they 'didn't want [the original] post to be ignored'. Although the adage, 'a problem shared is a problem halved' is something of a cliché, it seems very clear that people experiencing the beginnings of genetic illness, or a change in their genetic risk do need to connect with others who have some experience of their situation.

If we compare these very preliminary results with Carel's work, we can immediately see some similarities, and differences. Like Carel, many of these people felt unable to rely on their bodies, indicating a disharmony between the biological and lived body. Carel argues that this is caused by the body's malfunction, the existing physical symptoms. In many people with positive predictive test results there will be no physical symptoms, there is no failure in the objective body, although there is potential for failure in the future. The body remains the same, but the person's knowledge has changed. Does knowledge of a pre-existing weakness mean that the body is weak, or is the disruption caused by a change to the lived body rather than the biological body?

There are differences in relation to the social perception of illness. For Carel, the problem is that everything is out there for the world to consume. The physical problems mean that the illness cannot be ignored. For the genetics patient, this is reversed. The illness is hidden. There is no change in social perception because there is no catalyst for that change. This puts the onus on the patient to discuss their illness. If it is the case that solidarity and companionship is fundamentally important to coping with this sort of illness, then the hidden nature of the genetic condition may be even more of a burden than that suffered by someone with a physical problem, since solidarity may be much harder to find.[10]

Carel discusses the negative ways in which family relationships may be affected by chronic illness (Carel 2008 p. 58) citing examples of the need for care and support for the ill person. In the genetic predisposition situation, this is different again. While family members will no doubt experience similar concerns about care and support, they also have to deal with their own risks. This will compound the awkwardness that Carel notes in the interactions between family members, especially when we add in the possibility of relatives feeling guilty for worrying about themselves.

What Next?

Even this very preliminary exercise highlights some significant questions to do with the lived experience of genetic illness. As our understanding of genetic science improves, it is likely that many more of us will discover our predispositions to these illnesses. Existing philosophical work has not engaged with these questions, and our understanding of the experience of genetic illness is patchy at best. This problem needs rectification. Normative frameworks are likely to be impoverished if they are grounded in such a limited understanding of the issue. When we are talking about illness, where a person's experience is a fundamental part of the issue itself, we cannot afford to ignore this area of research or the phenomenological methodology illustrated here. If we want philosophy to be equipped to contribute to the problems of genetic illness, then phenomenological research is essential. It is only through understanding that we have any hope of offering answers.

Part Four

The Law, the Profession and Ethics

Chapter 12

Law at the Limits at the Limits of Life?

Richard Huxtable

Introduction

Decisions about whether to provide life support to critically ill children raise complex legal questions, spanning such areas as human rights,the criminal, civil, and family law. Nowadays, of course, such decisions fall under the broad umbrella of 'health care (or, more narrowly, medical) law'. A substantial collection of rulings (or jurisprudence) has developed in the English law, according to which seriously compromised lives need not be prolonged or saved. Yet, despite its heft and history, this is a body of cases that often fails to do that which we might legitimately expect of law: guide people, under a system of rules.

In this chapter, I describe in some detail a particularly difficult recent case, which came before the English courts on more than one occasion. The case involved the care of Charlotte Wyatt, who was born prematurely, and the question of whether (and to what extent) efforts should be made to sustain her existence. I will reflect on the law as it pertains to patients like Charlotte and reflect more generally on what we might expect from law, drawing on Roger Brownsword's helpful analysis of the 'rationality' of law. Applying this critical framework, it quickly becomes apparent that the English law in this area is seriously deficient. Much of the reason for this, I will suggest, rests on the legal officials' attempts to cling to competing – sometimes flatly contradictory – ethical commitments. Yet, this engagement with the ethical dimensions of the decisions is also commendable and arguably unavoidable, given the close relationship between ethics and law in this area. I close, therefore, with a plea for more open scrutiny of the values at stake in cases like these, particularly so that the law can best do that which it ought to do, that is, guide action. Although it will be apparent that my analysis specifically engages with the English law, there are undoubtedly issues here – concerning the interplay between law and ethics – which have far wider relevance.

At the Limits of Life: The Case of Charlotte Wyatt

Charlotte Wyatt was born on 21 October 2003, three months prematurely, with brain damage and severe problems with her lungs, heart and kidneys (see Jackson and Huxtable 2005). In the first 10 months of her life, Charlotte had to be resuscitated three times. The medical opinion was that she would be unlikely to see or hear, would not develop neurologically, and that her existence was, to her, intolerable. By September 2004, she was almost completely reliant on an 'oxygen box' in order to survive. The hospital Trust responsible for Charlotte's care approached Hedley J in the High Court for a declaration to the effect that it would be lawful to withhold artificial ventilation should Charlotte suffer a fourth crisis. Disagreement underlay the approach to court: Charlotte's parents, who were hoping for a 'miracle born of divine intervention' (*Portsmouth* 2004 para. 14), argued that she should be given the chance of life (perhaps even the chance to return home) and they made their position known in the national media.

At the first hearing in October 2004, Hedley J ordered that it would be lawful, in her best interests, for the paediatricians not to intubate and ventilate Charlotte, although CPAP (continuous positive airways pressure) could be administered in order to keep her airwaves open and ease her breathing, unless this caused her visible distress.

A few months later Hedley J was asked to stay these declarations, in view of perceived improvements in Charlotte's condition (*Portsmouth* 2005a). Her reliance on a 'head box', which supplied oxygen, had declined, and she could now spend periods outside it, albeit with the support of a breathing mask. Yet, despite such improvements, Hedley J felt that the orders could remain. He recorded the court's 'delight' at Charlotte's improvements and emphasized the strong presumption in favour of preserving life (*Portsmouth* 2005a, para. 16). However, the doctors' duty was still to act in the best interests of the child 'as and when any crisis might arise' and Charlotte's condition implied that she would be unlikely to 'survive such aggressive or invasive treatment' (*Portsmouth* 2005a para. 19). Indeed, he was concerned that the removal of the orders might encourage 'wholly false expectations' (ibid.).

The doctors did not expect Charlotte to survive the winter, and yet in April 2005 Hedley J was observing: 'in dealing with a child you can rarely be certain. Children do not stand still; they develop or regress' (*Re Wyatt* 2005 para. 3). Charlotte certainly seemed to have developed well: her oxygen requirements had further declined (to 50%) and she had become increasingly responsive to her environment and stimuli. Yet, the judge recognized also that 'her neurological condition remains about as bad as it could be' (*Re Wyatt* 2005 para. 6). Medical experts still maintained that Charlotte would not be able to withstand invasive efforts to deal with a respiratory crisis, given her severe chronic lung disease coupled now with malnutrition resulting from her inability to receive nourishment.

Hedley J was again persuaded that artificial ventilation ought not to be offered. The chances of such 'futile aggressive treatment' restoring her to her current condition after a crisis seemed slim and would most likely either threaten her chance of a peaceful death or return her to an 'intolerable' existence (*Re Wyatt* 2005 para.16). He decided that an 'anticipatory declaration' could be made, given the intractable (and seemingly 'volatile') nature of the disagreement between the parents and the health care team, and the fact that the nature of the crisis was 'fairly precisely anticipated' (*Re Wyatt* 2005 paras. 18, 21). He felt his declarations should nevertheless remain subject to review and, if or when the crisis came, it would remain the doctors' decision, in consultation with the Wyatts, to determine what ought or ought not to be done.

Charlotte was still alive in September 2005, when her parents went before the Court of Appeal, in which Hedley J's decisions were upheld. Delivering the judgement of the court, Wall LJ undertook an exhaustive examination of the law pertaining to best interests, with the aim of providing guidelines for future judges that were 'as clear and as simple as is consistent with the serious issues which they engage' (*Wyatt* 2005 para. 85). He felt it was 'nearly always a matter of regret' when cases like the present one had 'to be conducted in a courtroom, rather than a hospital or a consulting room' (*Wyatt* 2005 para. 86). When that happens, however, the test is indeed the best interests of the child. This test involves examining the issues 'from the assumed point of view of the patient' and working from the (rebuttable) presumption that life should be preserved (*Wyatt* 2005 para. 87). Medical, emotional and other welfare issues are included in the consideration and the court should undertake a balancing exercise, which might involve drawing up a 'balance sheet' of harms and benefits (*Wyatt* 2005 paras. 87, 89). Like Hedley J, the Court of Appeal felt that the notion of 'intolerability', while a 'valuable guide' to making the assessment, 'should not be seen either as a gloss on or a supplementary guide to best interests' (*Wyatt* 2005 para. 91).

Each case had to be decided on its specific facts and turning to this particular case, Wall LJ felt that Hedley J had proceeded appropriately in issuing 'permissive, not mandatory' declarations, which were amenable to review, and he noted that the Trust was also keeping its decision not to re-ventilate Charlotte under review and that this would be 'discussed with her parents before it is implemented' (*Wyatt* 2005 para. 114).

Wall LJ discouraged any belief that 'open-ended' declarations should be sought or that the court should be viewed as a 'general advice centre' since it is 'not the function of the court to oversee the treatment plan for a gravely ill child. That function is for the doctors in consultation with the child's parents... 'The court's function is to make a particular decision on a particular issue' (*Wyatt* 2005 para. 117). Although he disapproved of the Wyatts' occasionally 'less than helpful' conduct (such as reporting the doctors to the police for their perceived lack of care), he recognized the strain they were under and was encouraged by the news that their relationship with the Trust was improving. He hoped, then, that a treatment plan could be agreed at the next hearing (*Wyatt* 2005 para. 119).

The case thus returned to Hedley J, with the Trust now seeking a declaration to the effect that the doctors would have the final say in the event of a further dispute with the Wyatts. Heldey J felt that a 'novel' declaration of this sort was not required (*Portsmouth* 2005b para. 40). A doctor, he said, is obliged to act in the best interests of the patient, working 'in partnership with the parents' (*Portsmouth* 2005b para. 29). There may be occasions when parents and doctors disagree, on reasonable grounds, and in such situations the final decision might rightly be left with the parents. Yet, clinical judgement can comprise an intellectual dimension and a 'professional conscience, intuition or hunch', and the clinician cannot be compelled to act contrary to his or her conscience (although another professional might not be so troubled and might thus be willing to act) (*Portsmouth* 2005b para. 36). This, thought Hedley J, provided sufficient protection for Charlotte's doctors.

Four months later the case was back before Hedley J for another (and, for our purposes, final[1]) hearing (*Re Wyatt* 2006). Charlotte had been able to return home for visits but her condition had now deteriorated considerably: she had developed a cough and was apparently suffering from a viral infection. Intubation and ventilation looked likely to be the only available intervention if her condition continued to decline, and her parents (who had unfortunately separated) felt that this would lead her to recover, although the doctors unanimously felt it would be futile and contrary to her best interests. Hedley J issued another 'permissive and not mandatory' declaration that the doctors would be free to refrain from intubation and ventilation if, at the relevant time, they felt this would be appropriate in child's best interests (*Re Wyatt* 2006 para. 15). As of March 2009, Charlotte had reportedly been out of hospital for two years and living in foster care, since neither parent had been judged capable of meeting her needs, where she was learning to walk (Levin 2009).

Judging Law from Within

Charlotte Wyatt's case, while undeniably remarkable, is but one in a substantial body of jurisprudence, which considers whether life-sustaining measures can be withdrawn or withheld from a patient incapable (currently or perhaps ever) of expressing their views on the matter. 'The court's function is to make a particular decision on a particular issue' opined Wall LJ in the Court of Appeal. His colleagues have long insisted that the legal endeavour is precisely that: at the outset of his judgement in a landmark 2000 case before the English Court of Appeal, Ward LJ felt that it was 'important to stress the obvious. This court is a court of law, not of morals, and our task has been to find, and our duty is then to apply, the relevant principles of law to the situation before us – a situation which is quite unique' (*Re A* 2000 p. 969).

Leaving degrees of uniqueness to one side, Ward's statement is striking in its determination to separate law from ethics.[2] Cases like Charlotte's and, indeed, the one before Ward LJ (concerning the surgical separation of conjoined twins) certainly give rise to numerous legal questions. In the English law, for example, the position on the cessation of life-supporting treatment finds its roots in the criminal law but has grown to occupy a distinct field of health care law, gaining sustenance from family law, tort law and human rights law along the way. Even in its current incarnation, the legal position is pushed and pulled by such considerations as when life might (not) be ended, the human rights of patients, the scope of parental decision-making, and the duties owed by health care professionals. These certainly look like the sorts of issues on which law should take a stand. The problem, as we will see, is that on those occasions when the law has taken such a stand, it sometimes fails to do that which the law ought to do.

The idea that there are some things that the law ought to do – that there are legal virtues – requires some unpacking. To do this, we need to get within what Alastair MacIntyre would call the 'practice' known as law, where 'a practice' can be understood as:

> any coherent and complex form of socially established cooperative human activity through which goods internal to that form of activity are realized in the course of trying to achieve those standards of excellence

which are appropriate to, and partially definitive of, that form of activity, with the result that human powers to achieve excellence, and human conceptions of the ends and goods involved, are systematically extended (MacIntyre 2007 p. 187).

Lon Fuller illuminates the quest for the 'standards of excellence' associated with law by defining the legal endeavour as 'the enterprise of subjecting human conduct to the governance of rules' (Fuller 1969 p. 96). In a leading legal primer appropriately entitled *How to Do Things with Rules*, the authors define a rule as 'a general norm mandating or guiding conduct or action in a given type of situation' (Twining and Miers 1991 p. 131). While not alone in the endeavour, lawyers are, on this account, specialists in 'rule-handling'.

Roger Brownsword commends Fuller's neutral definition because it avoids begging any of the questions usually at stake in discussions about (for example) the connection between law and morality (Beyleveld and Brownsword 1994 p. 120). Brownsword sees particular principles of (practical) 'rationality' flowing from this concept of law (cf. Weber 1968). Law's central job is the regulation of human actions; rationality points the way to the 'best' actions, so, by definition, law ought to be rational in the ways Brownsword describes. He points specifically to three criteria: *formal* ('internal') rationality, which focuses on consistency in legal doctrine; *instrumental* ('system') rationality, which divides into *generic* and *specific* forms and concerns law's ability to fulfil its action-guiding goal; and *substantive ('norm')* rationality, in which the emphasis is on satisfying some justifying principle(s).

Formal rationality insists that legal doctrine should not be contradictory i.e. '*within a particular legal system* there should not be competing ground rules' (Adams and Brownsword 1995 p. 10, emphasis in original). Particular legal systems will fail this requirement where, for example, the legal officials adjudicate differently in materially similar cases. One might say (although Fuller would not: 1969 pp. 65, 69) that contradictory laws effectively cancel one another out, with the result that the law will say nothing about a practice about which it purports to say something. In the absence of such blatant inconsistency, formal rationality is also alert to 'less obvious contradictions screened from view by traditional compartments and categories' (Brownsword 1996 p. 152). The convenient creation of new labels, exceptions and sub-categories will not necessarily convince critics that consistency is restored.

Instrumental rationality focuses on the law's ability to guide action. Starting with the *generic* obligations, Brownsword borrows Fuller's eight requirements of the 'inner morality of law' (Fuller 1969 pp. 33–94). First, there must be rules – not specific edicts. The remaining seven requirements essentially insist that these rules must be capable of being followed (Radin 1989). Radin divides these latter requirements into 'know-ability' and 'perform-ability', where the first requires the rules to be promulgated, congruent, non-contradictory,[3] clear and constant, while the second insists that the rules must be prospective, possible of performance, and, again, not contradictory or incongruent.

As the label implies, *specific* instrumental rationality concerns the particular legal interventions chosen for specific situations (Brownsword 1993 pp. 255–256). If, for example, the aim is to prohibit, then something like the criminal law would be the right tool. Socio–legal enquiries into any 'gaps' between declared rules and official practices will help gauge the success of the chosen tool. Brownsword concludes that the generic and specific requirements 'must work together as a set of necessary and sufficient conditions for effective law' (Brownsword 1997 p. 32).

Brownsword's framework, so far, shares numerous features with accounts of the 'Rule of Law', from scholars including Dicey and Jennings, all the way up to Beale (1935), Raz (1977), Finnis (1986), Rawls (1972), and Dworkin (1985).[4] Whether such criteria are merely *formal* or procedural, or whether they entail or imply more *substantive* commitments is a recurrent theme in this literature (e.g. Hart 1965; Craig 1997). Up to this point there is good reason for siding with the former position: none of the requirements just outlined appear to commit law to what Fuller might term the governance of some 'external morality'. However, with his third criterion, Brownsword explicitly makes this connection. *Substantive* rationality, he argues, requires law to conform to a justifying end or principle, which he finds in the work of rationalist philosopher Alan Gewirth (1978). Gewirth claims to have derived the definitive moral principle, instructing us to respect the freedom and well-being of moral agents, from non-moral premises (essentially the fact of agency itself). In the final analysis, Brownsword would insist that the particular legal responses to a situation like Charlotte Wyatt's must fit within this normative framework (see Beyleveld and Brownsword 2001).

The Limits of Law at the Limits of Life?

To what extent does the law – and, by extension, the legal officials – measure up to the requirements associated with 'good' law in cases like Charlotte Wyatt's? It should come as little surprise that there are numerous failings in this difficult area. Let us start with those requirements pertaining to *instrumental* and *formal* rationality.

The primary obligation looks pretty straightforward: there must be rules. But consider again Wall LJ's observation that a judge must 'make a particular decision on a particular issue'. As Ward LJ further demonstrated, this insistence on the particularities of the individual case is a common mantra, which begins to suggest that this is a body of 'law' that fails at the first hurdle even to qualify as 'law'. Yet, the legal officials will surely retort that there is a rule in operation, which nowadays finds statutory expression in section 1 of the Children Act 1989: 'the child's welfare shall be the court's paramount consideration'. Unfortunately, here the problems mount up, since the rulings in which the denial of life-support from a critically ill infant is authorized in their best interests disclose a body of law that is not clear, or certain, or predictable.

The first thing to notice is the presence of distinct jurisdictions for dealing with cases like these: lawyers have been able to choose whether to seek an order under the Children Act 1989, where decisions will be made with reference to the 'welfare' of the child, or whether to invoke the inherent jurisdiction of the High Court, according to which the child is made a ward and decisions are taken in their 'best interests'. These might be little more than superficial differences, but they begin to suggest formal irrationality, in the sense that fine lines are sometimes drawn between cases, depending on the jurisdiction in which they are heard.

Such irrationality is arguably aggravated when one recognizes that there are many more cases involving the removal of life-support in which welfare and best interests considerations are heard in notably different ways. The courts have, for example, long drawn lines around that distinct body of cases involving patients in a persistent (or permanent) vegetative state whose clinically assisted nutrition and hydration is to be withdrawn (*Airedale v Bland* 1993). Such cases must come to court, which nowadays means coming before the Court of Protection, under the recently enacted Mental Capacity Act 2005. The judges in such cases are also required to consider the best interests of the patient, albeit, as this is understood under the terms of the 2005 Act. The same standards govern decisions (not) to treat incompetent adult patients who are not in a persistent vegetative state, although there is no requirement to bring these sorts of cases to court, even where the removal of treatment looks as likely to hasten death.

Even restricting ourselves to that body of case-law into which Charlotte Wyatt's sorry saga must be slotted, the failings of the English law are all too apparent. If, contrary to the earlier suggestion, we assume that the standards for welfare and best interests essentially amount to the same thing, then the question still arises: what is such a standard to mean? Wall LJ sought to shed some light on the matter in Charlotte's case:

> The judge must decide what is in the child's best interests. In making that decision, the welfare of the child is paramount, and the judge must look at the question from the assumed point of view of the patient. There is a strong presumption in favour of a course of action which will prolong life, but that presumption is not irrebuttable. The term 'best interests' encompasses medical, emotional, and all other welfare issues. The court must conduct a balancing exercise in which all the relevant factors are weighed and a helpful way of undertaking this exercise is to draw up a balance sheet... We urge caution in the application to children of factors relevant to the treatment of adults, although some general statements of principle plainly apply to both. (*Wyatt v Portsmouth Hospital NHS Trust* 2005 paras. 87 and 90, references excluded)

Superficially helpful, this statement nevertheless prompts a multitude of questions. How can a judge (or anyone, for that matter) examine the patient's interests from their assumed point of view, particularly when the patient has never been capable of expressing any views, thoughts or values? When can we say that the presumption in favour of life has been rebutted? And when such cases arise, are we saying that death is *in* the best interests of the patient or *not contrary to* their interests? What is the relative weight to be accorded to medical, emotional and 'other' welfare issues (whatever these latter are)? How is the balancing exercise to be conducted? What weight should be given to the different factors on each side of the see-saw? Is this a numbers game or is some form of qualitative weighting appropriate? In short, to use Radin's term, how 'know-able' is the concept of best interests?

Clear (or, to be a little kinder, clearer) answers to these sorts of questions are sorely needed if the law is to fulfil its aim of guiding people's behaviour through conformity to rules. The people in question are numerous: in the present context they include (at least) the parents and other loved ones of the patient, plus the health care professionals providing him or her with treatment and care. It is arguably not good enough that professionals can approach the courts in the hope of receiving guidance in the face of a fractious relationship between themselves and the patient's family, only to be told by the judge that any anticipatory decision would be 'fraught with danger', given the unpredictability of the situation (*R v Portsmouth* 1999 p. 910). One might sympathize with the difficulties inherent in an unpredictable clinical (and interpersonal) situation, but the lack of predictability in the law is less forgivable. Indeed, the deficiencies here are arguably illustrated by the simple fact that Charlotte Wyatt's plight returned so often to the courts. And once before the court, matters became little clearer: repeated references were made to the need to 'discuss' what should be done at any critical point, but what precisely was this to mean or require? To cite Radin again, how 'perform-able' is the resultant law in this area?

One can also detect inconsistency – even outright contradiction – in those cases that have been decided. Brownsword warned against rulings in which different results were reached in materially similar cases. The judges seem disinclined to permit direct comparisons, emphasizing the 'uniqueness' of cases, but comparisons are undoubtedly invited, especially in cases where the infants appeared to suffer from identical medical conditions. Most famously, there were the cases of John Pearson and baby Alexandra, in the early 1980s. Both had Down's syndrome with, it transpired, (remediable) complications. However, John Pearson's parents did not wish him to survive and he was allegedly left to die, which led to his paediatrician, Dr. Arthur, being charged with attempted murder (*Arthur* 1981). The doctor was acquitted of the crime. Critics expressed concern about the trial judge's apparent bias in the defendant's favour, given his deferential tone, sympathetic portrayal of what was legally (not) permitted, and apparent dismissal of the victim (described as 'the child' and even 'it') in his summing-up of the case for the jury (Huxtable 2007 pp. 110–111). But shortly before this trial, albeit, in the civil jurisdiction, the Court of Appeal had decided that baby Alexandra should have the life-saving operation, since her life was 'still so imponderable that it would be wrong for her to be condemned to die' (*Re B* 1981 p. 1424). No reference was made to the ruling in the judge's summing-up of the case against Dr Arthur.

Although Alexandra was to be given a chance at life, her judges nevertheless accepted that there was no obligation to prolong 'demonstrably awful' lives (ibid.). This concept accordingly initiated the series of cases, of which Charlotte Wyatt's is a more recent example. No longer does the spectre of the criminal law appear to hang over the doctors in cases like these. But even in the more modern cases one can detect tensions and conflicts. In 1998, artificial ventilation was removed from baby C, who had spinal muscular atrophy, despite the opposition of her Orthodox Jewish parents. Brown P acknowledged that the sanctity of life was 'vitally important' but confirmed that C's welfare was the paramount consideration (*Re C* 1998 p. 390). C had been expected to live no more than a couple of months. In 2006, doctors could not say whether baby M, who had the same condition, would die suddenly and soon or survive for a few years. Asked also to authorise the withdrawal of ventilation (again in the face of parental opposition), Holman J felt that the cases were distinguishable: M enjoyed greater awareness than C, and was (also unlike C) wholly reliant on the breathing support. He declined to authorize the proposed course, although he did accept that further life-saving interventions (like CPR) did not need to be offered, unless the doctors judged this to be appropriate at the relevant moment (*An NHS Trust v MB* 2006).

Beyond Law at the Limits of Life?

Cases like those of C and M will undoubtedly have their differences, particularly because disease courses will not always be identical. Yet, even if one views Holman J's efforts to distinguish the two cases in a sympathetic light, this is evidently an area of law blighted by uncertainty and irrationality. The reason for this is not difficult to detect, and it takes us back to Ward LJ's opening assertion that he was presiding over 'a court of law, not of morals'. That assertion rings false when one notices that Ward LJ thereafter spent a substantial portion of his judgement exploring and attempting to apply the principle of the sanctity of human life. In order to assess the adequacy of the fine lines that the legal officials seek to draw and the apparent irrationality that ensues, one cannot evade engagement with what Brownsword called 'substantive rationality'.

Not everyone will accept this point, which occupies a longstanding debate, as famously illustrated in the exchange between Hart (1963) and Devlin (1965) about the connection between law and morality. Sheila Mclean (2007a,b p. 196), for example, appears to separate the two domains and thinks that law will usually tend to trump 'ethics':

> irrespective of the ethical views of decision-makers – legal or medical – there are rules under which they must operate, like it or not. Whether or not they are based on moral obligations . . . they nonetheless are superior (in practical terms) to the outcome predicted by adherents to one ethical school of thought or another.

On this account, law trumps ethics in guiding action.

> Commitment to a particular ethical position may not be sufficient to guide practice, particularly when there are legal rules which differ from it or which require that other values are more important. Ethics and law are ultimately both interlinked and separate (McLean 2007a p. 198).

In the present context, the interlinked point is surely right. It is, after all, often the case in health care law that law simply cannot do its job without making reference to the ethical framework on which it rests. In short, legal arguments often must be supported by ethical justifications. In such circumstances, there is undoubtedly a case for examining closely these ethical underpinnings, not least in order to enable law to do its job as best as possible.

Here, an *immanent critique* can help in comparing how law would look if it sincerely and consistently observed the values it claims as its own with how it in fact looks (Pearson and Salter 1999). The problem in the area of law with which we have been concerned is that there are a variety of norms in competition. These norms can be mapped onto three rival accounts of the value of human life (Huxtable 2010).

First there is the *intrinsic* account of the value of life, according to which life should not intentionally be brought to a premature end, whether by action or omission. This account, closely associated with Judaeo-Christian (and particularly Roman Catholic) thought, does not insist on everything being done that could be done: disproportionate ('extraordinary') measures need not be taken, by which it is meant that 'futile' treatment can be withdrawn or withheld, as can measures which prove more burdensome than beneficial. Secondly, and in stark opposition to this account, there is the idea that life has only *instrumental* value, such that lives of great suffering, inability and even disability might well be truncated, perhaps even through intentional action. Thirdly, there is the idea that life has a *self-determined* value: this connects with the contemporary emphasis on respect for autonomy, which for some extends into parental autonomy and 'substituted judgements', in which the surrogate decision-maker puts him or herself in the position of the patient.

One glimpses each of these accounts in the jurisprudence pertaining to patients like Charlotte Wyatt. Ward LJ, for example, sought to emphasize the duty to protect life inherent in the intrinsic value of life, but his ultimate decision more closely resembled its rival, since it appeared to take a consequentialist approach, in which one 'normal' life saved outweighed the loss of one (or, perhaps, two) 'abnormal' life (or lives) (Huxtable 2000). One might nevertheless detect the ongoing pull of the sanctity of life in a decision like that of Holman J in the case of baby M. Or perhaps that decision is better read in terms of the instrumental value of life? Maybe, instead, Holman J drew the relevant 'quality of life' threshold at a higher point than his predecessor Brown P had in the case of baby C? One can certainly glimpse such thinking in the judges' occasional references to the idea of 'intolerable' lives. The authority – and thus autonomy – of parents is also a constant feature in cases like these, although no clear message necessarily emerges about the scope and limits of such authority, as Charlotte Wyatt's case so vividly illustrates.

It is not immediately apparent which of these rival groups of arguments ought to win out, if any, in the campaign to guide professionals, patients and parents in their daily health care transactions. Each set of arguments has considerable flaws, such that no single account should dominate at the expense of all others: they each, for example, are premised on contestable concepts, which can be used to defend some seriously questionable practices (see Huxtable 2007). Yet, equally, health care law is unlikely to get far if it does not go some distance towards recognizing each set of concerns. The problem, of course, is that in attempting to afford space to all such concerns, the law is undermined by tensions and occasionally blatant contradictions between its rules and their attempted applications.

Given all this, there might be merit in seeking to combine the relevant values, even along the lines of a compromise approach, according to which space is to be given to each of the principles, but each must also lose out (Huxtable 2007). An example of such an approach is where 'mercy killing' is kept subject to criminal censure but rules and practices mitigate against punitive application of the law in such cases (ibid.). Other situations in which core values come up against one another might warrant alternative accommodations. There is certainly merit in keeping such values under scrutiny. How we can best achieve this is itself a matter of some discussion, including again by Sheila McLean, who is critical of one such modern attempt. In a series of papers, McLean (2008) suggests that clinical ethics committees are not all that they could or should be, and that they would certainly benefit from a greater degree of formality. Indeed, she asks 'what and who are clinical ethics committees for?' (McLean 2007b).

I would suggest that clinical ethics committees can be a helpful supplement to the courts, especially in cases like Charlotte Wyatt's, where the conflict of values is so close to the (legal and clinical) surface, and few – including the judges themselves – believe that the courtroom is the best place to resolve matters (Ward Platt and Ward Platt 2005). I am, of course, not alone in thinking this: a recent committee convened by the Nuffield Council on Bioethics (2006) reached a similar conclusion. McLean (2008) doubts that clinical ethics committees are capable of supplanting law, at least as they are presently constituted in the UK. She has a point. However, I suspect that now is the time to consider how best to utilize such committees, in the face of what Doyal (1990) has described as moral and legal indeterminacy. Law – in the sense of specific rules, jurisdictions and legal principles – can only take us so far. Given the widespread indeterminacy in the cases we have surveyed, and the evident desire of parents and professionals to know what is expected of them, investing energy in the creation of fora in which the ethical dimensions of such difficult decisions can be aired openly and constructively is surely a worthwhile endeavour.

Conclusion

I began with a difficult case, from English law, concerning the (non-) treatment of a critically ill infant. I have, throughout this analysis, suggested that the law surrounding such cases is blighted by irrationality, as it is unclear, unpredictable and uncertain.[5] It will not escape notice that what I have not done is posit an answer to such cases that is itself clear, predictable and certain. Instead, I have suggested that there are important values questions at stake beneath these legal difficulties, to which more attention should now be devoted. One way in which this might be done, I suggest, is by reinvigorating clinical ethics support. As the label implies, a clinical ethics committee certainly sounds like the right place to consider the ethical dimensions to caring for patients like Charlotte Wyatt.

Many further issues emerge from this analysis, with regard to: committee composition and their members' training needs; the tools which enable these members to sift good ethical arguments from bad; the boundaries beyond which an ethical matter becomes a legal matter (and thus for the attention of a judge); and, the liability of such committees. Although more established elsewhere in the world, these committees are in their relative infancy in the UK and so this is the time to be considering these issues. There is certainly merit in encouraging a more open examination of the values at stake in decisions like those described in this chapter, and how those values can and should impact on and inform the law in ways that best enable it to fulfil its function. Given the plurality of people and positions at stake, this must be a shared endeavour, in which we seek to go beyond the current limits of law at the limits of life.[6]

Chapter 13

Bringing the Profession into Disrepute – an Ethical or Legal Issue?

Cliona McGovern

Introduction

It is probably safe to say that the healthcare profession is one that has the most ethical guidelines, regulations, declarations and laws written for it and about it. I do not mean just for doctors, I mean for the entirety of the healthcare professions put together. The amount of material regulating and guiding these professions is truly staggering. From the earliest beginnings of the ancient Pythagorean healer sects, throughout history and into our modern world, ethics and healthcare professions go hand in hand. This is an accepted truism and yet, in our modern world, something is happening. Slowly but surely our understanding of ethical behaviour is changing. There is a recognized emphasis on professionalism but for clarity on some important issues society has become increasingly reliant upon what is legal. This is a worrying development and is cause for concern. Have we now reached a point where ethics is seen as something that is dominated by law? Or worse, do we see ethics and professionalism as synonymous with the law? In this chapter I will explore this idea and use examples from modern healthcare that demonstrate the difference between what is ethical and legal and why this difference is important.

Before going further, we must ask ourselves the question: 'who is responsible for the continuing good practice and development of medicine itself – lawyers, philosophers or physicians?' This is neither a tricky question nor a rhetorical one as the answer is obvious; the responsibility lies with the physician. Who is responsible for ensuring the standards of good practice in medicine are maintained? Again, the responsibility lies with the physician and not with lawyers and philosophers. In most countries, a self-regulatory body that is legally recognized to be the authority on good practice, ethics and professionalism, governs the medical profession. It is, therefore, fair to say that medical doctors are responsible for what happens within their profession. This may appear to be somewhat an obvious thing to say, that doctors should be in charge of regulating the medical profession. But is that what we truly believe? Or rather, as a society, do we expect the courts to set out the rules for professional practice in medicine? In the discussion that follows, I examine a few cases where the courts have looked at this issue and have set out their own opinion on the matter.

Professionalism in Healthcare

As with all self-regulated professions, medicine itself has come in for much criticism in recent times for failing to regulate in a competent manner because they either do not know how to or do not have the powers to do so. In Ireland, during an investigation into the damaging practices of Dr Michael Neary,[1] Judge Maureen Harding Clark stated:

> The needs of the general public require that the professional bodies have the power and effective means at their disposal to monitor the competence of their members in order to ensure optimum patient care . . . There has to be a system for dealing with concerns at an early stage which does not have the stigma and ensuing upset of a complaint to the Medical Council or a high profile court action (Harding Clark 2006 pp. 339–340).

The incident under investigation at Our Lady of Lourdes Hospital, where peripartum hysterectomies were almost the rule rather than the exception to the rule, highlighted the difficulties that exist in stopping rogue practices or physicians. What happened with Neary's practice was, technically, not illegal[2] but it was certainly unethical and professionally incompetent. When the matter was brought to the attention of the relevant authorities, the Irish Hospital Consultants Association (IHCA) carried out an urgent peer review of Neary's practice in November 1998.

As set out in *Prendiville & Anor v Medical Council* in 2008, the Secretary General of the IHCA arranged for Neary to meet three consultants for the peer review.[3] The consultants were asked by the IHCA to submit a report on Neary within 72 hours. The report was prepared in an industrial relations context and was solely for the use of the IHCA in its dispute with the Health Board over Neary's suspension (Tottenham 1995, pp. 16–19). During the course of the review, it became evident to the three consultants that Neary carried out peripartum hysterectomies far more frequently than he should. Given the frequency of occurrence, the consultants obtained an undertaking from Neary that he would not perform any further peripartum hysterectomies without first seeking a supporting opinion from a second consultant. However, they deemed him safe to work and Neary was not suspended from practice.

When the findings of the official Lourdes Hospital Inquiry report were issued in January 2006, the Patient Focus group made a complaint to the Irish Medical Council's Fitness to Practise Committee (FPC) concerning the above three consultants (*Prendiville* para 134). The FPC found that the three consultants were guilty of professional misconduct because of their failure to recognize the seriousness of what had occurred with Neary's practice. The FPC stated that:[4]

> . . . professional misconduct as defined by Keane J in *O'Laoire v. The Medical Council* being conduct in connection with his profession in which the medical practitioner has seriously fallen short of the standards of conduct expected among medical practitioners (see Tottenham 1995 p. 17).

The FPC's decision gave the findings of facts but did not include the reasons for this finding. This is substantially different to the FPC findings on Neary, which included a report that ran to over 100 pages (Tottenham 1995 p. 17). When the Medical Council convened to consider the FPC's findings, it upheld the decision but did not consider any reports before coming to their conclusion. Additionally they did not impose any sanction on the three consultants. The Council then issued a press release that stated that the consultants were guilty of professional misconduct, but the press release did *not* mention the fact that no sanction had been imposed. Obviously, the consultants' professional and personal reputations were greatly damaged by this press release even though the Council had not sanctioned them in any way. In short, it appeared to the general public as though the Medical Council *had* issued a sanction as they were 'guilty of professional misconduct' but this was not the case.

Two of the consultants then sought to appeal the decision of the Medical Council but, in another twist, there were unable to do so. Under Part V of the Medical Practitioners Act 1978, it was not possible to appeal as no sanction had been imposed. Therefore, the consultants had no option but to request a judicial review, and sought an order of *certiorari*[5] of the Council's decision.

That case became the Prendiville case and in a detailed judgement, the findings of the Council were quashed (*Prendiville* para 176). The Court took a very dim view of what the Medical Council had done, and in quashing the decision of the Council and the FPC, the Court did not remit the matter back to the Medical Council (which is not what occurred in a similar case that I will discuss later). The Court ruled that the Medical Council was wrong in law and acted *ultra vires* in regarding itself bound by the decision of the FPC without looking for reasoned judgements or reports. As the Medical Council had solely confined itself to the question of penalty, the consultants were denied a process of natural justice. It was irrelevant to the Court whether the FPC was right or wrong in finding the consultants guilty of professional misconduct. The Court looked at the manner in which the investigation had been carried out and found the whole process to be flawed. Therefore, in quashing the findings, the Court 'wiped' the decision of the Council from the record.

Typically, when deciding if a doctor is negligent or their professional conduct is called into question, a test known as the 'expected standards test' is applied. This test, when dealing with cases of professional negligence, is known as the Bolam test,[6] and it means that if a doctor reaches the standard of a responsible body of medical opinion, she or he is not negligent, even if there is another body of opinion that might use a different medical technique. This expected standards test is clear and fair, and it is this standard that the FPC used when determining the outcome of the three consultants. They found that the expected standard would be for them to be aware of the negligent practices of Neary and request that he be suspended from practice. According to the FPC, the failure of the three consultants to do so meant they were guilty of professional misconduct.

However, in yet another twist to this case, the judge found that the FPC was wrong to use the expected standards test. The judge, referencing the various editions of the Irish Medical Council's *Guide to Ethical Conduct and Behaviour* stated that:

> . . . it is astonishing that in the five editions of the guide published by the Council between its creation in 1978 and the year 2004, nowhere in the definition of professional misconduct is the 'expected standards' test mentioned. It is not until the publication of the sixth edition in 2004, that it is to be found (*Prendiville* para 165).

Instead, the judge pointed out that the guidelines that were in force at the time the consultants were asked to carry out their report had a different standard, that of 'moral turpitude'. The judge then defined moral turpitude as:

> There is another standard of professional conduct which was referred to as the 'moral turpitude' standard. It can be defined as 'conduct which doctors of experience, competence and of good repute consider disgraceful or dishonourable' . . .

> In 1998 . . . in section A of the guide, which deals with conduct and behaviour, professional misconduct is described at para. 1.5. The definition is as follows:-
> 'Professional misconduct is conduct which doctors of experience, competence and good repute, upholding the fundamental aims of the profession, consider disgraceful or dishonourable' (*ibid.* para 162).

It is a perfect articulation of the 'moral turpitude' standard.

So, what is the difference between the expected standards test and the moral turpitude standard? It is this; the application of a moral turpitude standard does not require the court to hear from expert witnesses about what other people might do (unlike the expected standards test). It implies something about the person's state of mind when they carried out the action because they *knowingly* did something that was dishonourable. It can cover a wide range of things, from knowingly issuing a bad cheque, to driving without insurance, to theft and cheating. In the eyes of the law, moral turpitude is where someone knowingly acts in a dishonourable manner or in a way that is contrary to the considered norms of society or the morally acceptable standard.

In the Prendiville case, it is on this point (moral turpitude versus expected standards) that the FPC should have investigated the actions of the three consultants but they did not, choosing instead to follow the expected standards test. In my view, the decision to find the consultants guilty of professional misconduct was the right outcome but the manner in which that decision made was fundamentally flawed, thereby giving the court no option but to quash. It is irritating to know that the Council could have applied the moral turpitude standard as their own guidelines, articulated it properly, and could have investigated the matter more thoroughly than they did. Their failure to uphold their own guidelines meant that the three consultants, who could have stopped Neary much earlier than he was stopped, had no sanction imposed upon them.

It was not for the court to impose a sanction upon the consultants either. In fact, courts will not define the professional standards for *any* profession. This is an important point to keep in mind when thinking about the difference between law and ethics. There is a reason why there are ethical standards and legal standards. There is also a reason why the regulatory body is the correct institution to impose a sanction, no matter how strict that sanction may be such as striking someone off the register (a point which I will return to later).

The law itself recognizes that defining morality through the law is a dangerous, if not an impossible, task. For example, in a recent case in Ireland, the courts examined the question of moral turpitude when the issue of file sharing over the Internet was raised. Was a person, sitting at home in front of a computer, who knowingly downloaded copyrighted music over a file sharing service, guilty of moral turpitude? The court ruled that this question was beyond its remit saying that:

> It would undermine respect for the rule of law: for no one would know quite what the rule of law might be if it depended on attitudes forged through legal argument in individual cases as to what was acceptable conduct.[7]

In other words, if we relied on the law to define what was acceptable conduct, then the law would change from time to time, depending on what the attitudes of the society (or profession) would be. This completely undermines the respect for the rule of law as it would no longer rely on precedent and anything it had to say would solely depend on subjective attitudes. In our common law system, the law simply cannot operate in that manner. Therefore, for the professions, it is of prime importance that there be a regulatory body that will define what is, and what is not, an acceptable standard of ethical and professional practice. The law will not do this job for the professions but what it can do, as seen in the Prendiville case, is call the professions to account should they fail to uphold their own guidelines and procedures.

If doctors are to care for the health, healing and wellbeing of human beings (the main medical goals), then they *have* to be responsible for what they do and how they do it. It must be stated that those main medical goals are not determined by the whims of the society of the day either. The medical profession will always be responsible for maintaining our health and wellbeing, caring for us at all times. The responsibility for this good medical practice rests not only on each individual doctor but also on medical professional bodies. So, medical students and doctors who are already practising must know, uphold and understand their own ethical standards. More than this, they must recognize that ethical practice, and all the professional standards associated with it, including moral turpitude, is not something to be treated lightly. Acting in a professional manner is important as a failure to do so would bring the entire profession into disrepute.

Bringing the Profession into Disrepute

Another example of this failure to act in a professional manner is the, by now infamous, Bloodgate incident, where three professions[8] were thrown into disarray through varying degrees of professional misconduct and moral turpitude. For those unfamiliar with story, Bloodgate did not involve anything as serious as peripartum hysterectomies. It involved a game of rugby and the use of a capsule of fake blood.

In April 2009, the Heineken Cup[9] semi-final match took place between Leinster and Harlequins. A Harlequins player, Tom Williams, feigned injury by biting on a capsule of fake blood. Williams, with 'blood' evident on his face, then had to leave the field of play for a blood substitution. Only minutes remained in the game and Harlequins were trailing by one point. The player who was the goal-kicker, Nick Evans, had already been substituted earlier in the game and the only way to get him back on the field of play was through a blood substitution. The ruse was rumbled, thanks to the suspicions of the opposing team and the ubiquitous presence of numerous television cameras that caught Williams winking at his teammates as he walked off the field of play. An inquiry into the incident was launched almost immediately and the independent disciplinary committee of the European Rugby Cup (ERC) issued a finding that stated that:

> . . . this was a very serious offence and one that damaged the reputation of the tournament and of the rugby union, and accordingly the committee imposed a fine of 250,000 euros on Harlequins . . . The committee also suspended Mr Williams from playing rugby for a period of 12 months up to and including 19 July 2010(Rees 2009).

Despite this finding against the club and the player, the committee dismissed the misconduct complaints that were made against the Harlequins director of rugby, Dean Richards, and two members of the club's medical team, physiotherapist Stephen Brennan and Dr Wendy Chapman. The club, when the finding was released, issued a statement saying:

> Harlequins are both surprised and disappointed at today's decision by the ERC disciplinary committee to find Harlequins and Tom Williams guilty of misconduct – particularly so in the light of the acquittal of Dean Richards, Steph Brennan and Dr Wendy Chapman on similar or identical charges (Rees 2009).

I do not propose to detail here the entire sequence of events that occurred subsequent to that statement. Suffice to say that eventually, Richards, Chapman and Brennan were all eventually sanctioned and left the club. However, for the purposes of this discussion, it is interesting to examine what happened to the physiotherapist, Stephen Brennan, as his case focused on bringing his profession into disrepute.

The Physiotherapist

When the Bloodgate affair was investigated, it soon emerged that Brennan[10] played a significant part in the whole incident. The Health Professions Council[11] (HPC) ultimately laid a substantial number of charges against Brennan including the facts that he was the person who bought the fake blood capsules and had them ready in his bag to use when necessary.[12] In September 2010, considering the gravity of the charges against him, the HPC held their first Competence and Conduct Committee hearing, the result of which led to Brennan being stuck off the register. At the time, the Committee said:

> . . . the panel has been keenly aware that Mr Brennan's clinical ability is not in question. However, the dishonesty already referred to continued over a number of years and ended not as a result of his own volition, but only because of the player's subsequent admission . . . . The panel has no hesitation in finding that Mr Brennan's professional reputation remains stained. The finding of impairment of fitness to practise is required to demonstrate to the public and other health professionals that behaviour of this nature simply cannot be countenanced . . . . The striking-off order is a decision that is arrived at not only by a process of elimination, but also because it is the sanction the panel considers to be necessary for the public and other professionals to understand that behaviour of this sort is unacceptable (Rees 2009b).

Clearly, the Committee felt strongly that even though there was no issue with Brennan's clinical work, he had brought the physiotherapy profession into such disrepute, that they had no option but to strike him off the register. However, Brennan appealed that decision to the High Court, as was his right.[13] This appeal is only the second time since the HPC was established, that a case involving a physiotherapist appeared before the courts.[14] Given Brennan's very high profile status in the profession, the case and the subsequent decision was a landmark judgement.

The High Court case (*Brennan v. Health Professions Council*, 2011) focused on the argument that while Brennan acknowledged that his conduct had damaged the reputation of the profession, it did not merit a sanction as severe as a striking off. He did not appeal against the findings of misconduct, indeed he admitted almost all of the allegations against him, nor did he appeal against the conclusion that what he did impaired his fitness to practise as a physiotherapist.

Brennan's lawyers argued that 'one strike and you're out for good' was too harsh a penalty approach for someone whose clinical competency was not in question. In a similar case in the UK, the severity of penalty imposed by a regulatory body was considered when judgement was delivered on a solicitor who was appealing to his being struck off by the Law Society. In *Bolton v Law Society* (1994), Bingham said:

> . . . the consequence [of a striking off] for the individual and his family may be deeply unfortunate and unintended. But it does not make suspension the wrong order if it is otherwise right. *The reputation of the profession is more important than the fortunes of any individual member. Membership of a profession brings many benefits, but that is a part of the price* (emphasis mine).[15]

Even with the above comments in mind, the Court still ruled in Brennan's favour and the decision to strike him off the register was overturned. However, the Court remitted the matter to the HPC to hold another hearing into the incident and provide adequate reasons for their decision.[16] In deciding on remittal, the judge said that it was appropriate for the HPC's Competence and Conduct Committee to impose a sanction in this case because it is the body responsible for professional ethics (*Brennan* paras. 58 & 59). The point made by Ouseley J is a critical one and it is one that is frequently overlooked by governing bodies of most professions and institutions because they are 'in fear' of the law. Furthermore, it refers back to the moral turpitude discussion – it is not for the law to decide on professional ethics. As stated previously, the courts can (and do) call the professions to account should they fail to uphold their own guidelines but the court will *not* assume responsibility for defining what professional conduct and ethics should be (*ibid.*, at paras. 64 & 65).

As such, the reconstituted Committee hearing was held in May 2011. The Committee took serious note of what the Court had to say and also took into consideration the true remorse shown by Brennan.[17]

Mr Brennan is widely regarded as having learned a very hard lesson. All of the witnesses spoke of the series of lectures which Mr Brennan has given to other physiotherapists and health professionals about professional standards and medical ethics in the context of his experience at Harlequins Rugby Football Club and before the disciplinary and regulatory bodies.

Given all of the circumstances, which are detailed in the findings from the hearing, it was decided to issue Brennan with a caution that would remain on his file for five years. The importance of the decision from the court to refer the case back to the Committee proved one invaluable thing;

it is the profession itself who has the appropriate responsibility of investigating fitness to practice and all the surrounding areas that could bring the profession into disrepute. This responsibility does *not* lie with the legal profession. The law has its place – that of the courts – and it will ensure that the decision making process on professional sanctions is made by the appropriate body of people.

The Medical Student

You may ask, given this complex legal versus ethical debate, why must I drag the poor medical student into it? While the above cases have been well documented by the necessary regulatory bodies and by the courts, one of the more serious issues involving professional practice frequently involves medical students and a breach of patient consent and is hardly documented at all.

One of the most fundamental aspects of medical practice today is the informed patient; consent is paramount. Yet, it will come as a shock when it is realized that occasionally, once the patient is under anaesthetic in an operating theatre, medical students will carry out an intimate examination[18] on the patient without the patient ever knowing that such an examination had taken place or having consented to it. It is thought that obtaining patient consent to an intimate examination while under anaesthetic would result in few patients actually agreeing to the examination, thereby restricting the students' opportunities to learn.

In 2003, the BMJ published a study by Coldicott *et al.* (Coldicott 2003 pp. 97–99) that looked at this issue of medical students 'learning' by way of the intimate examination of anaesthetized patients. The authors surveyed 25 English medical schools and found that while most of them had established policies on teaching vaginal examinations, almost none had any guidelines for teaching rectal examinations (Coldicott 2003 p. 98). What is even more worrying is that students were able to compartmentalize what had happened. Though they knew that what they had done was wrong, it was, in their eyes, a breach of mere medical ethics and not (as they thought) a breach of law so it's 'not that big of a deal'.

In fact, as the article goes on to detail, in the absence of explicit consent, the *student* is liable to a legal charge of assault, just as they would be in every common law jurisdiction (Coldicott 2003 p. 99). If charges were brought against the Irish medical student, then it would be under the Non Fatal Offences Against The Person Act 1997 and, at a stretch, charges could also be brought under the Criminal Law (Rape) Act 1990. The consultant is not absolved from blame either as the examination took place under his or her direction, meaning changes can be brought against the consultant too. Does the fact that the patient was anaesthetized and never consented make the situation better? In light of what I have just said, I suggest not.

The authors in the BMJ study were concerned that of the 386 medical student responses to their survey, quite a lot of the comments from the students shifted responsibility for what had happened onto to supervising staff. Students said things like:

> 'You are expected to obey consultants by the fourth year. You can't refuse, and as doctors have to do uncomfortable things, so you just have to start early' (Fourth year student)
>
> 'You couldn't refuse comfortably. It would be very awkward, and you'd be made to feel inadequate and stupid' (Fourth year student)
>
> 'I was told in the second year that the best way to learn to do PRs [rectal examinations] was when the patient was under anaesthetic. That way they would never know' (Fourth year student) (Coldicott 2003 p. 99)

Of even greater concern to the authors were the replies which indicated, 'that some students continue to put the need to practise techniques above the need to practise ethically' (Coldicott 2003 p. 99). This study was published in 2003 and it caused quite a stir at the time but then it faded into the background. Recently, the issue has again been revisited by a different group of researchers and the authors expected to find that the situation had greatly improved. This was not the case. They report on their data and state that:

> Students are still being asked by senior clinicians to conduct intimate examinations without valid patient consent, sometimes in contexts in which multiple students examine one patient, and that most students still feel unable to refuse such requests. Furthermore, we suspect that this problem is prevalent across the clinical workplace, affecting medical schools across the UK and elsewhere (Rees and Monrouxe 2011 p. 262).

So, it is concerning that after the original study in 2003, things do not appear to have progressed very much by 2011. Even though some very high-profile cases had been heard by regulatory bodies and by the courts about informed consent, it still does not appear to have an impact in this aspect of medical training. It seems that in some cases, the anaesthetized patient is no more than a practice tool for students, and ethical practice is consigned to the lecture hall. The recent study also has quotations from medical students and they do not make for easy reading.

> 'heck it's gonna be on him [the consultant] anyway if anything comes of it – it's not my problem'
>
> 'If you're having your anus cut out then having someone's finger put in it anyway I just thought was an irrelevance basically so I have no qualms whatever about not having specifically consented her to allow me to do a rectal examination'
>
> '. . . but he was quite an aggressive surgeon anyway so I just went and did it' (Rees and Monrouxe 2011 p. 266)

However, the need for student to learn and the intimate examination of an anaesthetized patient need not be mutually exclusive. Firstly, as Coldicott already ascertained, most medical schools have policies for vaginal examinations (Coldicott *et al.* 2003 p. 98), therefore, it should be logical for them to have a policy for rectal examinations too. If a patient presents with a condition that requires an intimate examination (like prostrate cancer or cervical cancer), then an intimate examination is part of the operation. If students are going to be present in the theatre, then the patient needs to consent for the students to perform an examination under the surgeon's guidance. Just like any other operation, consent must be sought before proceeding. Obtaining consent for operations is part of what medical students do in the hospitals. They are supposed to meet with the patient and discuss what is going to happen. Sometimes they have this discussion with patients in conjunction with staff and sometimes they can do it on their own. The patient's consent is documented and where possible (i.e. not an emergency situation or situations where patient capacity is impaired) the patient signs the surgical consent form. *The Guide to Professional Ethics and Conduct* by the Irish Medical Council is clear on this point too:

> Consent given by the patient is the exercise of a voluntary choice; it is the giving of permission for the intervention to be carried out by competent professionals, where possible in an appropriate environment. You should explain the process in such a way as to ensure that patients do not feel that their consent is simply a formality or a signature on a page (p. 34 sec. 34.1).

However, failing to ask for patient consent because of fear of damaging sensibilities about intimate examinations is paternalistic medicine at its worst. If the examination is part of the operation then where is the issue? I suggest that the issue lies in intimate examinations being carried out when they are *not* part of the operation. Where, in all the discussion about professionalism, medical ethics and medical law, does it say that it is acceptable to conduct an examination, never mind an intimate examination, on a patient without their consent? It does not exist and in fact, it is quite the opposite.

There is hardly a medical student today who does not know about the concept of informed consent. They are introduced to it with a discussion that typically commences with the famous quote from Justice Cardozo from a case in 1914:

> Every human being of adult years and sound mind has a right to determine what shall be done with his own body; and a surgeon who performs an operation without his patient's consent commits an assault, for which he is liable in damages.[19]

Students are taught about medical ethics, about the informed consent of the patient and they are also taught about the aspects of medical law that they will need in their practice when they qualify. Why then does the following scenario still happen in medical schools? A medical student leaves the lecture hall after completing the course on medical ethics and medical law. She or he will, at some point, either attend or assist an operation. The patient is there, under anaesthetic, and the medical student is instructed by the surgeon to carry out an intimate examination. What should the student do; Refuse to do the examination? Ask the surgeon if consent has been obtained? Or do what she or he was told? In practice, almost all students will comply with the order to carry out the examination, even though they *know* it is wrong.

What is going *on* here? Why, after all the guidelines, the professional regulatory bodies and the teaching of medical ethics does the above situation still happen in our hospitals? Why, when people knowingly do something that is ethically wrong, the very definition of moral turpitude, do they still carry out the procedure? It gives no comfort that it has to be pointed out that performing an intimate examination without obtaining consent is, in fact, illegal. Making such a statement then 'prioritises' the law over good ethical and professional practice that even the courts, as discussed, do not believe is proper. It is disheartening to know that some medical students think medical ethics is useful for the big ethical issues like abortion, euthanasia, or for regurgitation at examinations but not much else.

The traditional medical ethics course focused on those big issues and invariably, lectures are delivered to students about the four sacrosanct principles; autonomy, beneficence, non-maleficence and justice. However, in the past number of years, the emphasis has changed. Now, medical schools tend to focus more on professionalism and introduce the professional and ethical standards to students as soon as they start their medical education. In a recent editorial in *The Lancet* the difficulties in educating student doctors about professionalism and ethics is discussed.

> Attitudes, values, and behaviours are recognised as being exceedingly difficult to assess, but these elusive qualities are arguably the most important that a doctor will possess . . . Effective facilitation of attitudinal learning is not instinctive for many medical educators. Therefore, to produce a professional doctor, there should also be more focus on ensuring that teachers think about how, as well as what, they teach (Horton, 2011 p. 1807).

The sentiments expressed in the editorial are not new – medical educators already know it is difficult to engage students about professionalism and medical ethics. Yet, the consequences of this failure to engage means that practices like intimate examination without consent continue in our hospitals. It still happens, despite all of the regulations, guidelines, documents and protocols used to educate the medical profession about something as simple as consent. It begs the question – do some doctors actually not want to know? In their minds perhaps 'doctor knows best' and those of us who persist in poking holes (no pun intended) in that theory should just go away.

In short, medical schools need to practice what they preach. If professionalism and good ethical practice is what they want from their graduates, then the schools must start by ensuring the students fully understand why they cannot examine someone without consent. Surely, this is not a difficult concept for medical educators to grasp? Clear professional guidelines about intimate examinations will help the student doctor when he or she is in the hospital. They have had their lectures, they understand the concept and now, armed with that knowledge, they can go and take a patient's consent for surgery. They can discuss what will happen to the patient in theatre without conveniently omitting the more awkward explanation about an intimate examination. Of course, if the patient is having his tonsils removed, then explaining an intimate examination in those circumstances will be very difficult indeed. I suggest that the patient should perhaps remove himself to safer, less proctology obsessed hospital forthwith. Or perhaps he could demonstrate some dexterous proctological skill of his own with a rolled up consent form and a passing surly surgeon.

Conclusion

As we have already seen, the profession itself defines and regulates good medical practice. One of the most fundamental principles of this professional practice is the trust between the doctor and patient. First and foremost, the doctor has a duty of care to the patient and the doctor is supposed to put the patient first and a medical student has the same duty of care to a patient that a fully qualified doctor does. We live in a society where we expect the professions, in whom we trust to act in our best interests, to behave without impunity. We trust that the professional regulatory bodies will define a set of good practice standards and hold those who breach them to account. We do not need to have an in-depth study to know how light-touch regulation failed in our banking and finance professions. No, we expect regulatory bodies to act fairly, appropriately, swiftly and when sanction is merited, that it is carried out. Furthermore, we also expect that when regulatory bodies fail in the duty to protect us, we expect the courts to then administer justice.

As educators, we trust that our students understand why medical ethics is important and how, armed with the knowledge of its importance, they would have the courage to say no when instructed to do something that they know is wrong. The medical student is part of the healthcare profession and they too, even though they are only students, have a responsibility to uphold the highest professional standards.

If the ultimate responsibility of medical ethics lies with the medical profession, as I believe it does, then it cannot be handed over to ethicists, philosophers, theologians, lawyers or to powerful social pressures. If this were to happen, and if this is what healthcare professionals allowed to happen, then they would become mere instruments of science. The 'practice' of caring for another human is reduced to a tool to do with what you wish. The courts acknowledge this and have specifically stated that it is not their function or right to define the ethical practice of another profession.

Therefore, for those who work in the healthcare professions, it is important to remember that the professional can only truly be a professional when, even under pressure, the patient comes first. If that situation is a peer review of a colleague's practice, then it is your duty to speak up should you find that practice to be dangerous, out-of-date or unlawful. If you are physiotherapist, then your duty is to your patients and your profession; the desire to win a game of rugby comes after your professional responsibilities. If you are a medical student and under pressure from a glowering surgeon, your own feelings of discomfort come after your primary responsibility to the anaesthetized patient before you. Granted, the medical student is in a particularly vulnerable situation as their future career prospects could rest with the surgeon who is currently directing him or her to do something unethical. This is where medical schools have a responsibility to ensure that such a situation cannot arise and, if it does, that the student has the support of the school.

Medical ethics is not always about the big issues such as euthanasia and neither is medical law. Increasingly, the issues before regulatory bodies involve moral turpitude problems like lies, cheating, cover-ups and deceit. These are the day-to-day medico ethical problems that bring healthcare professions into disrepute and destroy the increasingly fragile trust that we, as a society, place in these professions. Professional ethics and the law work together, each responsible for different facets, but each with a power to correct and sanction where necessary. For the some of those in the professions, it is time to realize that a breach of ethics is 'that big of a deal'. A failure to comply with the ethical standards that are set out by the profession can result in a striking-off, the most serious consequence for any healthcare professional. Regulatory bodies will hold healthcare professionals to account for bringing the profession into disrepute, and, should that investigation need to be questioned, so will the courts.

Chapter 14

Conscientious Objection in Medicine

Mark Wicclair

Many doctor–patient encounters are routine and do not generate ethical conflicts or challenges. One important type of exception can occur when providing a lawful medical good or service, such as emergency contraception (EC), abortion, sterilization, forgoing medically provided nutrition and hydration, or palliative sedation to unconsciousness, is contrary to a physician's conscience. Such encounters can present difficult ethical dilemmas for physicians. On the one hand, as physicians they have obligations toward their patients. On the other hand, as moral agents, they feel obligated to follow their conscience. An important ethical question, then, is whether conscience-based refusals to provide a medical good or service are compatible with physicians' professional obligations.

Are Conscience-Based Refusals Compatible with a Physician's Professional Obligations?

Answers to this question range over a continuum (Cantor and Baum 2004; Wicclair 2011). At one extreme, there is an answer aptly termed the 'incompatibility thesis', which maintains that conscience-based refusals to provide legal goods and services within the scope of a physician's competence are incompatible with her professional obligations. At the other extreme, there is an answer aptly labelled 'conscience absolutism', which maintains that physicians should be exempted from performing *any* actions that are contrary to their conscience. Finally, in between these two extremes, there is an answer aptly designated 'compromise', which maintains that conscience-based refusals can be consistent with a physician's professional obligations, but only if specified ethical constraints are satisfied.

The incompatibility thesis

A statement by Julian Savulescu, although he subsequently qualifies it, expresses the incompatibility thesis: 'If people are not prepared to offer legally permitted, efficient, and beneficial care to a patient because it conflicts with their values, they should not be doctors' (Savulescu 2006 p. 294). A *New York Times* editorial conveys a similar view in relation to pharmacists: 'Any pharmacist who cannot dispense medicines lawfully prescribed by a doctor should find another line of work' (Anonymous 2005 p. 12). In defense of the incompatibility thesis, it can be argued that physicians who refuse to provide a good or service for reasons of conscience put their interests above the patients' interests and thereby fail to fulfil their professional obligations (Rhodes 2006).

In response, it can be claimed that there are limits to the sacrifices and burdens that physicians are obligated to make for patients. For example, primary care physicians are not obligated to make house calls or schedule appointments at night and on weekends; and if they make arrangements for a temporary substitute in order to take vacations, it is not a violation of their obligation to patients. In short, it can be argued that the incompatibility thesis is based on an indefensible conception of the professional obligations of physicians (Wicclair 2008 and Wicclair 2011).

Additional objections to the incompatibility thesis include: 1) Physicians can specialize and limit their practice without violating their professional obligations. For example, an orthopaedic surgeon who specializes in bunion surgery is not subject to the charge that refusing to perform other types of foot surgery or hip replacement surgery is a violation of her professional obligations. Hence, it is not always incompatible with a physician's professional obligations to limit the goods and services within the scope of her competence that she offers to patients. 2) Whereas advocates of the incompatibility thesis treat practitioners exclusively as physicians with professional obligations, doctors are also moral agents with their own personal ethical beliefs. 3) Advocates of the incompatibility thesis give insufficient weight to reasons for protecting the exercise of conscience. 4) If the primary aim is to protect patients, a compromise approach can provide adequate protection.

Conscience absolutism

The Pharmacists for Life International Model Conscience Clause is a paradigm of conscience absolutism:

> The rights of conscience of any person being a duly licensed pharmacist, who shall object on personal, ethical, moral or religious grounds to the performance of *any act* in the normal course of professional performance or dispensing, shall be respected. Further, such a refusal to perform *any act* or the *omission of any act* based on such a claim of conscience, shall not form the basis for any claim for damages or any recriminatory or discriminatory action against such a person (emphasis added).[1]

The corresponding view in relation to medicine holds that physicians never should be required to act against their conscience. In support of conscience absolutism it can be maintained that permitting physicians to follow their conscience is necessary to avoid moral complicity and protect their moral integrity (Pellegrino 2002).[2]

Objections to conscience absolutism include the following: 1) There are degrees of complicity (Sulmasy 2008), and the conception of moral complicity underlying conscience absolutism is too simplistic. 2) Conscience absolutism is incompatible with the professional obligations of physicians and other health care professionals (Brock 2008; Cantor and Baum 2004; Charo 2005). 3) Not requiring anything of health care professionals who receive conscience-based exemptions from providing a good or service that is against their conscience is inconsistent with the alternative service requirement that applies to conscientious objectors to military service (LaFollette and LaFollette 2007).

Of the three objections, the second may be the strongest. The first objection may depend on a controversial conception of moral complicity. Moreover, it might rely on a conception of complicity that is contrary to a physician's conscience. The third objection can be challenged on the grounds that the alternative service requirement for conscientious objectors to military service is not a suitable model for conscience-based refusals by physicians. Specifically, it can be maintained that unlike conscientious objectors who are exempted from military service, physicians who receive conscience-based accommodations already provide a wide range of 'alternate' services that are no less demanding, burdensome, or risky than those that they refuse to provide. Moreover, physicians who received conscience-based exemptions can minimize increased burdens for colleagues by agreeing to take on some of their more unpleasant tasks.

Compromise

As presented by Dan Brock, the 'conventional compromise' permits physicians and pharmacists to refuse to provide a service or product that is against their conscience only if the following three conditions are satisfied:

1. The physician/pharmacist informs the patient/customer about the service/product if it is medically relevant to their medical condition;
2. The physician/pharmacist refers the patient/customer to another professional willing and able to provide the service/product;
3. The referral does not impose an unreasonable burden on the patient/customer (Brock 2008 p. 194).

The conventional compromise is subject to the criticism that, depending on the circumstances, it may impose restrictions on the exercise of conscience beyond those needed to adequately protect patients and fulfil a physician's professional obligations (Wicclair 2011).

Ethical Constraints on the Exercise of Conscience

Although neither extreme is acceptable, there is a grain of truth in conscience absolutism as well as the incompatibility thesis. Conscience absolutism captures an important connection between the exercise of conscience and moral integrity: To maintain her moral integrity, a physician must refrain from performing actions that are against her conscience (i.e. actions that violate her core moral beliefs). Thus, the exercise of conscience is essential to maintaining and protecting a physician's moral integrity.

There are several reasons for permitting physicians to maintain and protect their moral integrity. First, moral integrity can be an essential component of a doctor's conception of a good or meaningful life. In this respect, moral integrity has intrinsic worth or value to the individual physician. Second, a loss of moral integrity can be devastating. It can result in strong feelings of guilt, remorse, and shame as well as loss of self-respect. Third, it might be claimed that when a failure to accommodate core moral beliefs gives rise to a loss of moral integrity, the result can be a general decline in a person's moral character, which is particularly undesirable in physicians. Finally, it can be claimed that moral integrity generally has intrinsic worth or value. That is, it might be asserted that, *having* core moral beliefs that are associated with one's self-conception and a *disposition* to act in accordance with them (to act conscientiously) are intrinsically valuable and worthy of respect. To be sure, insofar as moral integrity can involve a commitment to any ethical or religious beliefs, it does not guarantee ethically acceptable behaviour. However, it is not implausible to claim that similar to courage and honesty, which also can serve immoral ends and produce undesirable consequences, moral integrity is a moral virtue.

The incompatibility thesis captures the important point that physicians have an obligation to care for and protect their patients. This obligation is acknowledged in professional codes. For example, addressing UK physicians, the General Medical Council's *Good Medical Practice: Duties of a Doctor* identifies a duty to '[m]ake the care of your patient your first concern' and a duty to '[p]rotect and promote the health of patients and the public' (GMC 2006). The American Medical Association's (AMA) *Code of Medical Ethics* asserts that doctors in the United States have a similar obligation: 'The relationship between patient and physician is based on trust and gives rise to physicians' ethical obligations to place patients' welfare above their own self-interest and above obligations to other groups, and to advocate for their patients' welfare' (Council on Ethical and Judicial Affairs 2010 p. 374).

The obligation of physicians to place patients' welfare above their own self-interest or to make the care of patients their 'first concern' is a characteristic of a fiduciary relationship. Several reasons can be given for using the fiduciary model to conceptualize the physician–patient relationship. One appeals to the end(s) of medicine (See for example Pellegrino and Thomasma 1981 and Pellegrino 1993). It is claimed that the end(s) of medicine (e.g., healing), together with the vulnerability and dependence of patients and the distinctive knowledge, skills, and power of physicians, supports the fiduciary model. From a contractarian perspective, it can be claimed that the fiduciary model represents a reasonable choice for doctors and patients from behind a 'veil of ignorance' that prevents them from knowing whether they are doctors or patients. Alternatively, a social contract account can be used to support the fiduciary model. It can be claimed that: 1) the duty to place patients' welfare above physicians' self-interest is part of an agreement between society and the medical profession, and 2) when physicians enter the profession, they (implicitly or explicitly) agree to place patients' welfare above their own self-interest (See for example Rhodes 2006). Finally, the fiduciary model can be supported by reciprocity- or gratitude-based accounts of the physician–patient relationship (See for example May 1975). That is, it can be claimed that the duties associated with the fiduciary model are based on the benefits, rights, and privileges that physicians enjoy as members of the medical profession.

The ethical constraints of the 'conventional compromise' capture the important point that neither extreme is justified. However, the following more nuanced and context-dependent ethical constraints, expressed as physician obligations, adequately protect patients without unnecessarily limiting physicians' exercise of conscience: 1) an obligation to protect patients from excessive harm or burdens; 2) an obligation to assure that patients have an *opportunity* to learn about lawful and medically suitable options; 3) an obligation to be *willing* to refer and/or facilitate a transfer. Beyond these modified ethical constraints, physicians with conscience-based objections have two additional obligations to patients: 4) an obligation to give timely notification to patients, and 5) an obligation to eschew invidious discrimination. These five ethical constraints represent a reasonable compromise between physicians' interest in moral integrity and patients' interest in timely and convenient access to medical goods and services.[3]

Protecting patients from excessive harms and burdens

Depending on the circumstances, when physicians refuse to provide a good or service that is against their conscience, patients can experience substantial harm and/or burdens. Exposing patients to such harms/burdens is contrary to a physician's obligation to put his patients first. Unfortunately, there is no bright line separating harms and burdens that are excessive from those that are not. One point is clear, however: It is inconsistent with the obligation to put patients first to maintain that no matter how substantial the harms or burdens that a patient might experience, they cannot be excessive when they are the result of the exercise of a physician's conscience. Moreover, despite the absence of a 'bright line' separating harms/burdens that are excessive from those that are not, there are clear cases toward either end of the excessive/non-excessive continuum.

The seriousness of a patient's condition and the urgency of the patient's need for the refused good or service are among the factors affecting the magnitude of harms and burdens that will result from a conscience-based refusal. For example, the potential harm of a refusal to provide an emergency laparotomy generally is greater than the potential harm of a refusal to provide an elective first trimester abortion or fertility services.[4] The following are examples of situations in which refusing to provide a medical good or service can result in excessive harm/burdens: 1) The only surgeon on call at a community hospital refuses to perform an emergency laparotomy for a patient with a ruptured ectopic pregnancy. If surgery is not performed immediately, there is a high risk of death or serious permanent injury (e.g., infertility or incontinence). 2) A victim of a brutal sexual assault is transported by ambulance to the emer-gency department of the only hospital within 50 miles. Consistent with the hospital's religion-based policy against dispensing emergency contraception (EC) and the personal moral beliefs of physicians with hospital privileges, none of the physicians are willing to provide it. Due to the severity of the patient's injuries, it is impossible to transfer her to another hospital without exposing her to a significantly increased risk of mortality or morbidity. As a result of the refusal to provide EC, the rape victim does not receive it within the time-frame of its effectiveness.[5] 3) Marilee, a two-year-old who underwent unsuccessful treatment for cancer, is suffering from multiple organ failure and is near death. She is in the hospital's paediatric intensive care unit (PICU) and is being kept alive by various life support measures, including mechanical ventilation, vasopressors, and dialysis. In view of Marilee's grim prognosis, her parents request that all life-prolonging measures be discontinued, and they want her care to be limited to 'comfort measures'. The only paediatric intensivist who is currently on service in the PICU refuses to honor their request for reasons of conscience. Marilee dies four days later, and her parents believe that as a result of the physician's conscience-based refusal, she endured unnecessary pain and suffering.

As these examples indicate, whether or not a conscience-based refusal is likely to result in excessive harm/burdens is in part a function of the availability of other physicians to provide the good or service in a timely manner. For example, if another surgeon had been available to perform an emergency laparotomy for the patient with a ruptured ectopic pregnancy, the surgeon's refusal to perform it would not have exposed the patient to a risk of excessive harm. Similarly, if Marilee could have been transferred to an intensivist who did not have a conscience-based objection to withdrawing life support, the objecting intensivist could have exercised her conscience without violating her obligation to avoid exposing Marilee to excessive harm/burdens.

Location can be significant. When a physician in a large metropolitan area refuses to provide a good or service for reasons of conscience, there are likely to be other physicians who are willing and able to provide it. However, in small rural communities, the number of physicians may be very limited and many may have similar ethical or religious beliefs. In such communities, when a physician refuses to provide a good or service for reasons of conscience, residents may have to travel substantial distances at considerable inconvenience and expense to receive the good or service, and they may also experience substantial delays.

Even though there is no bright line separating harms/burdens that are excessive and those that are not, the constraint against excessive harm/burdens is not inconsequential. First, it serves to prohibit clear instances of excessive harms/burdens. Second, it serves as a reminder that physicians who have conscience-based objections to providing a good or service also have obligations to patients that may not be ignored. Third, it expresses the important point that determining whether or not the exercise of conscience is ethically justified is in part context dependent.

Assuring patients have an opportunity to learn about medically suitable options

Despite the Internet and various other resources available to the general public, patients often are dependent on physicians for reliable information about goods and services that will meet their health needs and interests. This dependence is a basis for the conventional compromise's disclosure requirement, which obligates physicians to inform patients about a good or service they refuse to provide 'if it is medically relevant to their medical condition' (Brock 2008 p. 194). Arguably, the obligation to give priority to patients' interests would justify this requirement if, whenever a physician has a conscience-based objection to providing a good or service, patients would not know that it is a clinically suitable option for them unless the physician informs them. However, this generalization does not always hold.

To be sure, there are situations in which disclosure by a physician with a conscience-based objection is essential. A modified version of the case of Marilee, the two-year-old who was dying after unsuccessful cancer treatment, provides an example. Suppose her parents are unaware of the option to discontinue life support and limit Marilee's care to comfort measures. The paediatric intensivist who is currently responsible for Marilee's medical management has a conscience-based objection to withdrawing life support and, for this reason, fails to inform Marilee's parents of that option. After Marilee's death, her parents learn that withdrawing life support and limiting care to 'comfort measures' is accepted medical practice in cases such as their daughter's. They are very upset when they realize that by withholding information from them, the physician exposed Marilee to suffering that they could and would have prevented. As this case illustrates, patients and surrogate decision-makers may depend on physicians for information about end-of-life options, such as withdrawing mechanical ventilation, discontinuing dialysis, forgoing medically supplied nutrition and hydration, and providing palliative sedation to unconsciousness (sedating terminally ill patients to unconsciousness until death). Patients and surrogates also may rely on physicians for reassurance that these and other options are *acceptable* (or at least, that they are lawful, accepted by the medical profession, and chosen by many patients and surrogates in similar circumstances).

Reliance on physicians for information about acceptable options is not limited to end of life decision-making. For example, several studies have reported that many women are either unaware of EC or lack sufficient understanding to use it effectively.[6] Accordingly, rape victims may rely on emergency department physicians for timely information about the availability of medication to prevent pregnancy.

If a physician has a conscience-based objection to providing x, a legal good or service within the scope of his professional competence, what are the physician's disclosure obligations to patients for whom x is a clinically suitable option (or to their surrogates, for whom x is a clinically suitable option)? To answer this question, consider Dr. Warren, who has a conscience-based objection to x, and Ms. Steinhart, one of Dr. Warren's patients for whom x is a clinically suitable option. To satisfy his obligation to give priority to Ms. Steinhart's interests, Dr. Warren has an obligation to ascertain whether Ms. Steinhart knows that x is one of her options. A request by Ms. Steinhart for x would obviously indicate that she has this knowledge. However, to prevent Ms. Steinhart from mistakenly inferring that x is not a clinically suitable option for her, Dr. Warren should clearly communicate that his refusal to provide x is for conscience-based reasons and not because x is medically unsuitable. If Ms. Steinhart does not request x, it is not sufficient for Dr. Warren to state that there is an option that he cannot disclose because doing so is against his conscience. Such a statement does not give Ms. Steinhart sufficient guidance to determine whether the unidentified option has enough potential value to warrant trying to find out what it is. Moreover, if time is of the essence, Ms. Steinhart may not learn about x soon enough. In addition, Ms. Steinhart might continue to worry that she has not identified *the* option that Dr. Warren would not disclose. Accordingly, if Dr. Warren determines that Ms. Steinhart is not aware of x, he is obligated to help her acquire information about it. Dr. Warren can satisfy this obligation by informing Ms. Steinhart about x. Alternatively, it can suffice to tell Ms. Steinhart that there is a clinically suitable option that he cannot disclose for reasons of conscience and offer to arrange for her to see another physician who will provide information about it.

This illustration of the obligations of physicians with conscience-based objections to disclosing clinically suitable options features a patient, Ms. Steinhart, who is able to make decisions for herself. When patients lack decision-making capacity, physicians have corresponding disclosure obligations to surrogates.

This qualified contextual specification of an obligation to disclose clinically suitable options can provide greater protection of conscience than the blanket disclosure requirement of the conventional compromise, but only when its exercise does not fail to satisfy the obligation to assure that patients have a timely opportunity to acquire an understanding of all of their clinically suitable options.

A willingness to refer and/or facilitate a transfer

When physicians refuse to provide a good or service for reasons of conscience, there is a continuum of follow-up behaviour that can affect patient access significantly. At one end of the continuum, doctors can actively help patients obtain access to the good or service by facilitating a transfer to a physician who is willing and able to provide it. At the other end of the continuum, physicians can actively thwart or impede a patient's access to it by, for example, obstructing or delaying transfer to another physician. Referral to a physician who is willing and able to provide the good or service, a requirement associated with the conventional compromise, falls somewhere between the two extremes.

There are two obvious reasons for a constraint against actively blocking or impeding a patient's access to a legal and clinically suitable good or service. First, such behaviour is inconsistent with the obligation to protect and promote the health of patients. Second, that behaviour also fails to respect patient autonomy.[7] Physicians who actively block or impede patient access may only intend to avoid *their complicity* in the perceived wrong-doing of others (e.g., patients and/or other physicians). However, another possible aim is to prevent *the patient* from engaging in behaviour that is contrary to the physician's ethical or religious beliefs. If someone believes that an action is seriously immoral, it is understandable if she also is committed to preventing others from performing the action. Nevertheless, it generally is inappropriate for physicians to exploit their professional gate-keeping power and authority to impose their ethical or religious beliefs on patients who do not accept them. Moreover, even if a physician's intent is only to avoid *her own complicity* in a perceived moral wrong, the effect can be to impose her ethical or religious beliefs on a patient who does not accept those beliefs, which is inconsistent with respect for patient autonomy.

Typically, accommodations for conscientious objectors enable individuals to refuse to perform actions contrary to their conscience, such as military service, abortions, prescribing and dispensing EC, and providing palliative sedation. The point is to allow individuals to refrain from performing actions against their conscience and preserve their moral integrity. However permitting y to refrain from acting against y's conscience is not to be confused with enabling y to prevent z from performing legal actions that are contrary to y's, but not z's, ethical or religious beliefs.

When physicians refuse to provide a good or service for reasons of conscience, patients sometimes do not need referrals in order to obtain access to it. However, sometimes patients do need assistance to secure timely and convenient access. In such situations, refusing to assist a patient is inconsistent with the obligation to protect and promote the health of patients. Depending on the situation, such assistance can involve providing a referral or facilitating a transfer to a physician who is willing and able to provide the good or service.

Frank Chervenak and Laurence McCullough identify a situation in which they claim an obligation to protect patients from harm requires referral. They maintain that in view of 'the sorry history of incompetently performed abortions, physicians with a conscience-based objection to abortion have an obligation to offer patients, who are considering the procedure, information about 'responsible health care organizations such as Planned Parenthood' (Chervenak and McCullough 2008 p. 232.e2). This obligation is said to derive from a physician's 'fiduciary responsibility to protect the patient from loss of future fertility, health, or even her life' (*ibid.*).

Although their assessment of the risk of harm without referral might be questioned, it is hardly debatable that a failure to provide a referral, if it is necessary, to protect patients from such substantial dangers is contrary to a physician's professional obligations.

When a transfer of care to another physician is required to accommodate a conscience-based refusal, hospital patients generally cannot be expected to assume the responsibility for effectuating it. For example, if, for reasons of conscience, an attending physician refuses to write a Do Not Resuscitate (DNR) order for a competent patient who has requested it, the patient cannot be expected to arrange for a transfer to a physician who is willing to write a DNR order. Even if the patient has a family who can assist, it is inappropriate to place on them the responsibility and burden of arranging a transfer. They may lack sufficient practical knowledge, and they already are likely to be under considerable emotional stress and strain. It may be acceptable for the attending physician to delegate to other members of the health care team, the specific measures required to effectuate a transfer. However, it is the attending physician's responsibility to set in motion the process and to assure that a smooth and timely transfer takes place. Withdrawing from the case without discharging this responsibility is tantamount to patient abandonment.

Sometimes, when physicians refuse to provide a medical good or service for reasons of conscience, it may not be feasible to determine reliably whether a patient needs assistance to secure access to it that is safe, effective, timely, and not excessively burdensome. However, to protect patients adequately and minimize the risk that physicians will fail to fulfil their professional obligations, the default position is an obligation to *offer* to refer or facilitate a transfer. That is, unless the physician has good reason to believe that the patient does not need the physician's assistance to secure access that is safe, effective, timely, and not excessively burdensome, the physician has an obligation to *offer* to refer and/or facilitate a transfer. Like the foregoing specification of the obligation to disclose clinically suitable options, this is a qualified contextual specification of the obligation to refer and/or facilitate. It, too, can provide greater protection of conscience than the conventional compromise, but only when the exercise of conscience is consistent with a physician's professional obligations.

Giving timely notification to patients

The timing of patient notification can significantly affect the impact on patients of conscience-based refusals. Patients are prone to be especially vulnerable and dependent at times when they need medical treatment. To minimize the negative impact on patients, whenever feasible and apt, physicians should provide advance notice to patients of conscience-based objections. Generally, if physicians have a conscience-based objection to providing a good or service within the scope of their competence, they should not wait until it becomes a clinically suitable option to inform patients that they cannot provide it. Physicians may be able to minimize harms and burdens by giving (prospective) patients an opportunity to learn about their conscience-based objections during the initial appointment. It is then that finding another doctor is the least upsetting and distressing. Advance notification can also maximize a patient's opportunity to establish a relationship with another physician—one who has no conscience-based objection to providing a good or service that the patient someday may want.

For example, if Dr. Crasswell, an obstetrician–gynaecologist, has a conscience-based objection to performing abortions, she should make this information available to prospective patients. Women who know that Dr. Crasswell has a conscience-based objection to performing abortions may decide to select an obstetrician–gynaecologist who will provide the service if and when they decide to have an abortion. Decisions about abortion can be highly charged emotionally, and learning about Dr. Crasswell's abortion policy before a prospective patient develops a relationship with her can prevent the unnecessary additional irritation, annoyance, and stress of having to change doctors. Prospective patients may be reluctant to inquire about Dr. Crasswell's willingness to perform abortions, or it may not be a concern to them at the time of their first appointment. Hence, it is Dr. Crasswell's responsibility to give patients and prospective patients an opportunity to find out that she is unwilling to perform abortions. She might, for example, give patients and prospective patients pamphlets listing services that she does and does not provide.

Advance notification can be particularly important in relation to end-of-life decisions. Suppose, for example, that Dr. Brown has a conscience-based objection to withdrawing medically provided nutrition and hydration (MPNH). Waiting to communicate her objection to withdrawing MPNH until patients or family remembers request it can add unnecessary stress and anxiety to an already highly tense and emotionally charged situation. Transferring the care of patients can be especially traumatic in end-of-life situations. Since patients and/or family members may be especially vulnerable, refusing to continue caring for a patient if he or members of his family insist on withdrawing MPNH may be perceived as abandonment and may evoke feelings of self-doubt, anger, and/or resentment. Dr. Brown can prevent making bad situations worse by providing timely advance notification of her conscience-based objection to withdrawing MPNH. However, advance notification has to be exercised with care so as to minimize the risk of causing rather than preventing unnecessary distress. For example, if Dr. Brown informs a patient who presents with a suspicious lump in her breast that she is conscientiously opposed to forgoing MPNH, the patient is likely to mistakenly infer that she has terminal cancer and is dying. Dr. Brown might appropriately disclose her conscience-based objection to withdrawing MPNH in the context of a routine discussion of advance directives with her patients.

Circumstances may not warrant advance notification. However, when it is feasible and apt, it can reduce harm/burdens and enable patients to select and establish relationships with physicians who are willing to provide goods and services that are consistent with their health needs and preferences.

Eschewing invidious discrimination

There is an important distinction between two types of conscience-based refusals: 1) refusals based on a belief that a medical *good* or *service* (e.g., EC or abortion) is unethical and 2) refusals to provide a good or service to *specified classes of patients* (e.g., Blacks, Muslims, lesbian women, gay men, and unmarried women). The second type of refusal is based on invidious discrimination. It is a settled view—one based on defensible and widely shared conceptions of justice, equality, dignity, and respect—that invidious discrimination is ethically wrong. Even if it is conscience-based (i.e., rooted in core moral beliefs), no accommodation of such invidious discrimination is warranted.

Consistent with this general ethical prohibition of invidious discrimination, professional codes typically prohibit it. For example, Paragraph 7 of the General Medical Council's *Good Medical Practice: Duties of a Doctor* cautions doctors: 'You must not unfairly discriminate against them [patients] by allowing your personal views to affect adversely your professional relationship with them or the treatment you provide or arrange'. An explanatory note about 'personal views' states: 'This includes your views about a patient's age, colour, culture, disability, ethnic or national origin, gender, lifestyle, marital or parental status, race, religion or beliefs, sex, sexual orientation, or social or economic status' (GMC 2006). The American Medical Association's *Code of Medical Ethics* includes a similar prohibition of invidious discrimination: 'physicians who offer their services to the public may not decline to accept patients because of race, colour, religion, national origin, sexual orientation, gender identity or any other basis that would constitute invidious discrimination' (Council on Ethical and Judicial Affairs 2010 p. 349).

Fertility doctors who refuse to provide services to lesbian women violate the obligation to eschew invidious discrimination if their refusal is based on the patient's sexual orientation. However, the following actual case illustrates how difficult it can be to determine the basis of denial of fertility services to lesbian women.[8]

Guadalupe Benitez, a lesbian, wanted to become pregnant and requested fertility treatments from Dr. Christine Brody, an obstetrician–gynaecologist at the North Coast Women's Care Medical Group in San Diego, California. At the first appointment Dr. Brody told Ms. Benitez that she would be willing to provide some fertility treatments, but if they failed, she would not provide intrauterine insemination (IUI), a medical procedure that involves threading a catheter through the patient's cervix to enable semen to be inserted directly into the uterus. Dr. Brody stated that it would be contrary to her religious beliefs to perform the procedure *on Ms. Benitez.*

One of the factual issues in dispute is Dr. Brody's reason for refusing to perform IUI on Ms. Benitez. Whereas Dr. Brody alleges that she told Ms. Benitez she would not perform it on an *unmarried* woman, Ms. Benitez claims that Dr. Brody told her that she would not perform IUI on a *lesbian.* From the perspective of California law at the time, this is an important distinction. Ms. Benitez sued Dr. Brody, NorthCoast, and another physician for violating the Unruh Civil Rights Act (CA Civ. Code § 51 [a]–[f]).[9] Although it was subsequently amended to prohibit both types of discrimination, at the time it prohibited discrimination based on sexual orientation, but it did not prohibit discrimination on the basis of marital status. However, denying services on the basis of a patient's marital status is no less an instance of invidious discrimination than a denial of services based on a patient's sexual orientation.

Had Dr. Brody refused to provide *any* fertility services to Ms. Benitez, it is reasonable to assume that the refusal was based on her sexual orientation or marital status. However, Dr. Brody provided some fertility services to Ms. Benitez. Unfortunately, no public documents about the case explain why Dr. Brody was willing to help Ms. Benitez conceive but drew the line at IUI. Thus, her reason for refusing to provide IUI is unknown. What is clear, however, is that it is inconsistent with the obligation to eschew invidious discrimination to refuse to provide services solely on the basis of a patient's sexual orientation or marital status.

As in the Benitez case, it may be difficult to determine whether conscience-based refusals involve invidious discrimination. First, such determinations require ethical judgements about what constitutes *invidious* discrimination, and in some cases controversial ethical assumptions may be needed to justify those judgements. Second, such determinations can require ascertaining intentions and reasons, and such determinations can be elusive. Nevertheless, when conscience-based refusals are based on invidious discrimination, they are incompatible with a physician's professional obligations.

Conclusion

Physicians have an interest in moral integrity, and patients have an interest in timely and convenient access to medical goods and services. Since maintaining moral integrity may require physicians to refuse to provide goods and services, these two sets of interests can clash. Hence, it is necessary to find a reasonable compromise between them. A reasonable compromise is to permit conscience-based refusals if physicians satisfy each of the following obligations: 1) an obligation to protect patients from excessive harm or burdens; 2) an obligation to assure that patients have an opportunity to learn about medically suitable options; 3) an obligation to be willing to refer and/or facilitate a transfer; 4) an obligation to give timely notification to patients; and 5) an obligation to eschew invidious discrimination.

Chapter 15

Clinical and Ethical Judgement

Julian C. Hughes and Steve Ramplin

Introduction

The judgement that someone should start a tablet to lower cholesterol (a statin) is not a simple thing, although it may be quickly made. What we shall argue in this chapter is that clinical judgements inevitably reflect forms of life: a whole set of beliefs and other judgements need to be in place in order to accept that the statin is required. In the pages that follow we shall present an argument along the lines below.

1. Clinical judgements are, at one and the same time, ethical judgements.
2. At first blush, it would seem that the art of making clinical judgements is acquired in the medical school, but good clinical judgement is one example of good judgement in general. How do we, therefore, acquire any capacity for judgement?
3. Judgements are normative: there are criteria of correctness.
4. Understanding the normativity of clinical judgements is to understand the normativity of ethical judgements.
5. Clinical judgements do not always feel like ethical judgements, they often feel procedural: we just act like this.
6. Basing judgements in practices also shows us something about the nature of normativity.
7. Practices are reflective of broader forms of life or ways of being-in-the-world.
8. So, when we acquire practices in medical school, we cannot solely be learning algorithms.
9. There are things that have to be presumed even for learning to take place. This gestures at the possibility of tacit knowledge underpinning our judgements. As is also the case in the acquisition of good judgement in general.
10. Although facts can be taught, what must also be in place to make clinical judgements is experience of the right sort.

Clinical Judgements are Ethical Judgements

While it is obvious that a decision not to resuscitate someone is clearly an ethical decision, it is worth noting too that even the decision to prescribe a simple analgesic, e.g. paracetamol, involves ethical judgement. At the very least, prescribing drugs involves the use of resources. Of course, there may be a host of other ethical considerations that emerge in connection with particular decisions, however seemingly trivial, which also require judgements of an ethical nature to be made. For instance, perhaps in this case it is known that the person once took an overdose of paracetamol. Hence, there may be several different types of ethical judgement required, by which we mean judgements about what is right or wrong, good or bad.

There is, however, more to it. It is not just that we can always think of an ethical dimension to medical practice. It is rather that clinical judgements are *at one and the same time* ethical judgements. It is not that we make the clinical judgement and then afterwards can ponder on the ethical implications. Of course we can do this; but the further point is that the clinical judgement is also, inherently, an ethical judgement.

This reflects a deep vein of thought about values in medical practice (Fulford 1989). There is a tendency to consider facts and values as separate things. Indeed, the tendency is to think that unless we keep facts and values distinct we are likely to run into error. This is understandable, because it would be an error to think of certain value judgements as factual judgements. It would be an error, for instance, to allow ageism to be thought of as having a factual basis. Nevertheless, in healthcare – that is, in the actual practice of healthcare – there are no facts without values. A simple date of birth is a fact, but the moment it is stated in the context of actual healthcare it starts to have evaluative implications. Facts are value-laden we might say. In the field of psychiatry, the evaluative nature of many judgements is obvious, including judgements about diagnosis (Sadler 2004). But evaluative decisions have to be made in every branch of medicine and the need for this is increasing, not decreasing; hence the need for values-based medicine (VBM), which we have discussed above in Chapter 6 (and see Fulford 2004), as the complement to evidence-based medicine.

The value-laden nature of facts in healthcare practice means, that clinical judgements cannot escape being, at one and the same time (i.e. inherently), ethical judgements. A moral question can always be raised in connection with any healthcare decision: was this the (ethically) right thing to do? Moreover, the evaluative concerns will always be different because of differing circumstances, even if many of the facts are the same. The moral question (about what is good and what bad) is, therefore, always particular: is it a good thing to give *this* man the statin *now* given his history and current cholesterol level? We should note, therefore, two important and related elements: the particularity and the context of the case. But enough has been said to establish that clinical judgements are, at one and the same time, ethical judgements. For, of treatment decisions it can always be questioned whether the particular judgement was right or wrong. Furthermore, diagnosis itself involves some form of value judgement (e.g. when is a wheeze asthma?), which in turn raises questions about what we consider to be good or bad states. On the whole, we are likely to accept that suffering is a bad thing, whereas the restoration of health is regarded as a good thing.

Acquiring Clinical Judgement

It would seem reasonable to assume that the ability to make clinical judgements is acquired during medical training. To make clinical judgements requires knowledge of certain facts, which include facts about likely outcomes. These facts are acquired in medical school. Given that medical school involves not only factual learning but also the acquisition of clinical skills, the idea that clinical judgements are taught in medical schools does not, at first blush, seem outlandish. The judgement that someone has left ventricular failure is a matter of experience, but this is backed up by knowledge of the facts about physiology and, more precisely, abnormal physiology.

A little more needs to be said about the sort of experience of which we speak. It could be said that left ventricular failure, in a straightforward case, is not too difficult to recognize. To the extent to which this is true, it could be argued that some diagnoses can be made on the basis of just a few acquired facts, without much experience. But experience is, nevertheless, required for more complicated cases. To anticipate, we want to argue further that, even in the straightforward (easy) cases, there has to be a background against which judgements are made. And, we wish to say, this background is inevitably value-laden: it is in part constituted by immanent judgements about what is good (e.g. normality or the restoration of health) and what is bad (e.g. suffering and loss of functioning).

If it is true, however, that clinical judgements are, at the same time, ethical judgements, then it must also be true that acquiring the knowledge and skill to make clinical judgements involves, at the same time, some form of ethical insight attached to those clinical judgements. There are two points. First, clinical judgements themselves involve evaluative decision-making at a variety of levels. Secondly, good clinical judgement is, in any case, an example of a broader type of good judgement. Clinical judgements might immediately involve ethical decisions (e.g. is it right to give this expensive treatment?); but, as exemplars of general good judgement, clinical judgements might also, more radically, reflect background evaluative features to do with, for instance, what is right or wrong, good or bad, for human beings as such.

How, then, is all this acquired at medical school? We shall initially consider two possibilities, which can be likened to how medical ethics used to be taught and to how it might now be taught.

First, it could be that students are taught the clinical facts about left ventricular failure so they are in a position to make clinical judgements, but they are not taught anything in connection with the surrounding ethical judgements. It is presumed that these have been or will be acquired from elsewhere. We might consider, at least in the context of medical schools in the United Kingdom (UK) that this was how clinical education proceeded say 25 years ago. There was no formal teaching of medical ethics. This did not mean that clinical judgements were unethical, because people either already had ethical codes of conduct or they were learning them through a process of osmosis: by observation of their teachers, by experience, and so forth.

A second possibility is that students are taught in the clinic that these are the signs of left ventricular failure. At some other point, in the lecture theatre, there is teaching about possibly related ethical judgements: about when it is right to start treatment, about why some treatments might be unethical, and about issues surrounding consent. The judgement that treatment is required, even if this would be universally agreed, is still one that draws upon a background understanding that the restoration of function is a good thing; and there may be conditions where treatment is only really warranted when symptoms and signs have reached a certain level of severity. Judging the type of treatment might involve the principle of non-maleficence and, thus, in the case of heart failure, avoidance of angiotensin-converting enzyme (ACE) inhibitors where there is significant renal disease. Ethical issues in connection with consent might involve judgements about capacity or coercion.

Students are now expected to acquire some formal understanding of medical ethics, where this tends to mean that ethical dilemmas can be discussed in terms of the four principles (Beauchamp and Childress 2009):

autonomy, beneficence, non-maleficence and justice. There are reasons to favour osmosis over formal learning and vice versa. The current situation can be considered better than the previous situation on the grounds that, at least, there is now a greater awareness of the need to pursue critical thinking in connection with clinical judgements. Furthermore, as science has progressed, the need for critical thinking about complex ethical dilemmas has increased.

There is, however, a third possibility – and it may be that, where teaching and learning are at their best, this has always occurred – which is that the art of clinical and ethical judgement-making are acquired simultaneously. In other words, the one does not happen without the other. This would seem to be the better way if, as we have argued, clinical judgements must truly be, at one and the same time, ethical judgements. It is important to note that our suggestion is not that two things are occurring, but solely one. The judgements are, at one and the same time, clinical and ethical. Of course, they can sometimes be separated. Also, however, the normative nature of the judgements will just entail that their ethical or moral nature is inherent.

This takes us back to the point about good clinical judgement being one example of good judgement in general. Although it will sometimes be the case that the ethical components of a clinical judgement can be conceived in an overt way as separate from the more routine factual or biomedical aspects of the judgement, there will be times when the moral component seems buried. For example it may be taken for granted that the aim is to restore health and that this needs doing in this case. We want to say that the background that makes this possible is good judgement generally. And then the question is whether being at medical school in any way contributes to such general good judgement. It will not in certain cases be irrelevant. But our suggestion is that the capacity for acquiring judgement of any sort ultimately rests on a way of engaging with the world.

The Normativity of Judgement

The next move, then, is to see that the judgements with which we are concerned are normative. In other words, there are criteria of correctness: not just anything will do. Statins should only be given under certain circumstances. Meningococcal meningitis should be treated with benzylpenicillin. These clinical judgements conform to norms of practice according to which there are right and wrong answers. It would not do for the doctor to give the wrong antibiotic before sending the person with suspected meningococcal disease to hospital.

But we may wish to note that clinical judgements can change. Perhaps one day *Neisseria meningitides*, which causes meningococcal meningitis, will become resistant to benzylpenicillin. In this sense, clinical judgements are contingent. In which case, however, perhaps they are not normative. We might think, that is, that if the rightness or wrongness of the decision changes, the normative nature of the judgement is undermined. But this is because we are thinking of judgements in general, not particular clinical judgements made in precise concrete circumstances.

The concern is understandable, but only when looking at clinical judgements in a particular way, from the outside one might say. Now consider what it is like actually to make a clinical judgement. The moment we decide that this is meningococcal meningitis, we are constrained to act in certain ways: we should give benzylpenicillin and arrange immediate emergency admission to hospital. This constraint is normative. We might make uncertain judgements: we have a suspicion about the child although there is nothing more than the signs of an upper respiratory tract infection. But if this is the case, there will be different ways in which we are normatively constrained: we should give the parents very careful advice about what to do if they are worried or if a rash were to start to appear; we should plan to review the child later on the same day. Whatever the judgement (that things are certain or uncertain), as we leave the child, we should have the feeling that, under these particular circumstances, in this context, we have done the right thing, albeit with a degree of uncertainty. There remain innumerable contingencies. Clinical judgements involve dealing with these sometimes unknown possibilities. The point is, however, there are normative constraints (criteria of correctness) concerning what we *ought* (ethically) to do. In this case the ethical 'ought' is not simply a matter of a duty to be obeyed, but of a deeper engagement with the world. If the clinical judgements are uncertain, the normative constraints will accommodate this uncertainty.

From the inside, therefore, there is something normative about our clinical judgements, which seems to reflect their nature as, at one and the same time, ethical judgements. This normativity does not feel as if it is something added on to the clinical judgement, it is embedded. The presence of a purpuric rash and the associated diagnosis of meningitis carries with it, inherently, the requirement to act in certain ways. In real situations, therefore, the clinical judgement will carry with it an imperative to act in particular ways and not others. This is what the normativity amounts to and our suggestion is that this reflects the nature of clinical judgements as being, at one and the same time, ethical judgements. At the very least, then, the experience of making clinical decisions does not mirror the experience of being taught ethics in medical school. This does not establish that the way medical ethics is taught is wrong, just that the lack of simultaneity in terms of learning about clinical and ethical judgements is not like the experience of making such judgements.

Understanding Normativity

One possible proposition, in order to understand normativity, is that we should seek to understand ethical judgements, because these seem to be the feature of clinical judgements that are normatively constraining. But our view is that this gets things round the wrong way. Instead, we wish to suggest, it is more useful to understand clinical judgements in order to understand the normativity of ethical judgements.

Going to medical school (and recall that we are using this to epitomize medical education as a whole, in other words the lifelong experience of medical practice) is a hugely complex psychological and sociological affair (Sinclair 1997). Students must be turned into medical professionals, with all that this entails in terms of knowledge, skill, confidence, compassion, empathy, and so forth, the exact mixture of which will depend on prior temperament and the specialty being chosen.

The end result is someone who can practise well and safely. There is an undoubted process of socialization by which the student acquires the norms and values of the profession. Of course, individuals may well decide to reject certain norms and norms change for a variety of reasons (consider, for instance, changes in the way that doctors dress). But some things have to be accepted. Doctors cannot ignore the importance of confidentiality as a professional principle. There are certain ways to examine a patient. There are practice guidelines to be followed. The end result of the process of socialization, however, is that students become practitioners. They enter medical practice. Moreover, there are accepted patterns of practice (Hughes 2006). We engage with patients in certain ways and not others, we treat them according to established practices.

In other words, there is a clear sense in which becoming a clinical practitioner is to acquire certain forms of normative constraint; and, as part of this, mastering the ability to make clinical judgements is simply to imbibe normative principles. To understand the normativity of ethical judgements, we should look to the normativity of clinical judgements. This reflects two lines of thought: first, in any case, clinical judgements are, at one and the same time, ethical judgements; and, secondly, it is the clinical judgements that we have before us.

The first line of thought, remember, is really that there is no gap between the clinical and the ethical. There is no dichotomy: they are one and the same thing. The second line of thought might suggest that ethics is separate from clinical practice, but not if practice is inherently ethical.

The Procedural Nature of Clinical Judgements

One thing that might contribute to wrong thinking is the idea that ethics is, in some sense, hidden. The idea comes from the possible thought that, whereas you can see the result of a clinical judgement (the statin is prescribed), an ethical judgement is hidden. You would have to ask someone about the nature of any ethical judgements they have made. You cannot see a person's ethics – think, for instance, of a case where the person's intentions seem to be key – whereas you can see clinical practice and, thereby, judge their clinical judgements.

But, actually, it seems reasonable to argue that you can see whether what a person thinks is ethical: you can simply look at what they do. We can judge by their actions that so-and-so has a tendency to be paternalistic, but that his colleague shows the virtue of compassion and that someone else clearly ranks respect for autonomy as a high priority. We are what we do. To observe a doctor's clinical practice (albeit anyone can be deceitful) is one way to learn something about his or her moral inclinations (i.e. inclinations about what is good or what bad), which will underpin the doctor's ethical judgements (i.e. concerning what is right or wrong).

Becoming a doctor partly means that, under particular circumstances, we shall act in ways that conform to a particular pattern of practice. In response to a high blood cholesterol result, doctors will consider using a statin. There may be reasons to pause, depending on the patient's views and values, or depending on other physical factors (e.g. poor renal function or hypothyroidism), but on the whole the practice is to treat raised cholesterol. In a large number of cases, however, doctors would act without any great ratiocination, speculation or contemplation. In a sense, then, many clinical judgements stem from and reflect a rather procedural approach. It is not always evident to the actor that what is done, as part of a procedure, is none the less a reflection of implicit ethical judgements. But actions are not just actions. They are themselves embedded in a set of values and evaluative concerns.

Evaluative clinical judgements are iteratively developed across generations and reflect changing attitudes in society (e.g. increased patient expectations), developments in terms of professional codes (e.g., in the UK, the General Medical Council's duties of a doctor as set out in *Good Medical Practice* (GMC 2006)) and scientific progress (e.g. the development of statins themselves). The way in which scientific progress increases choice and has an effect on evaluative judgements brings to mind VBM. Values will inevitably have an impact on clinical judgement. When values are relatively shared – as they might be concerning the initial treatment of meningitis for example – judgements are relatively straightforward. Clinical judgements become more complex in the face of conflicting values: abortion, euthanasia, many psychiatric disorders and even in connection with the use of statins (Ravnskov *et al.* 2006). Perhaps clinical judgements are more straightforward when values are shared because the ethical judgements seem less contentious. However, where values are diverse, clinical judgements are more complex partly because the ethical judgements involved are much more noticeable. This is precisely because the relevant and disputed values are on the surface owing to their diversity.

But, whether values are on the surface or hidden (because shared), actions are not just actions, because they incorporate evaluative decisions. It is not that there is a one-to-one correspondence between actions and ethical judgements. Also, people can be deceitful. But, on the whole, the particular action, in the context of similar such actions, gives a glimpse of the person's ethical outlook, which is why we might wish to start by looking at clinical practice and clinical judgements.

The Nature of Normativity

By looking at clinical judgements we can start to say something about the nature of normativity. Once again, we need to keep in mind that we are talking about actual cases where there are particular circumstances and a specific context. For one thing, then, normativity is immanent. Here is the practice of reducing cardiovascular risk factors, one element of which is to check the blood cholesterol level. If it is high, the standard practice is to try to lower it. There are a number of ways to do this, but a standard practice, under the right, particular and specific circumstances, is to prescribe a statin. This is – under the right circumstances – what we must do as part of the practice. It is normatively constrained that we should consider this. There are criteria of correctness that say this is the thing to do. It does not follow that we shall always prescribe a statin, because this would depend on the particular and specific circumstances. It may be that there is an unacceptable risk of muscle toxicity; or perhaps the patient wishes to try harder with a change of diet. But, under the right circumstances, it is correct to offer and discuss a statin and to prescribe one. The criteria of correctness are immanent in the practice. The normativity is an inherent feature of this aspect of medical practice. To modify cardiovascular risk factors simply means to do this sort of thing. In other words, we can also say that the normative nature of clinical judgements is constitutive of clinical practice in this regard. We can see, therefore, that clinical judgements demonstrate normativity as an immanent and constitutive feature. Nor can it be reduced to something else. It has a special quality aside from any factual or procedural points that might be made about the practice. The normativity that is immanent in and constitutive of the clinical judgement that a statin is required cannot be reduced to some other feature of the judgement. Normativity, in summary, is clearly seen to be immanent, constitutive and irreducible (Hughes 2011).

Practices Reflect Broader Forms of Life

So far we have argued that clinical judgements are, at one and the same time, ethical judgements and that they are normative in the sense that there are criteria of correctness relevant to such judgements. We have further said that the normativity of clinical judgements reflects the normativity of ethical judgements, but in order to understand this normativity we are better off looking at the concrete, real examples of clinical judgement because it is in these actual, specific circumstances that we see the immanent, constitutive and irreducible nature of normativity.

Normativity is to be found in practices. So it seems sensible to consider practices a little further. The first point we wish to make is that practices are patterned. They are not random. If, however, this sounds as though practices are somewhat pedestrian, we need to recognise that our lives are made up of practices and are deeply patterned in a layered manner (Hughes 2006). Patterns of practice, therefore, can be found not solely in professional practice, but more broadly in our social lives. Indeed, patterns of practice are essential for the meaningful use of language. The issues around language, meaning and judgement are complex (Luntley 2003). If we briefly consider the extent to which language is itself a practice, this opens up the discussion to some of the insights of Ludwig Wittgenstein. According to Wittgenstein, language reflects forms of life. The background point Wittgenstein was making was that we understand a language when we grasp how to use it. In other words, it is not a matter of a theoretical mastery of a language from the outside. It is a matter of grasping a practice from the inside, as it were: a matter of being as we are, people who act like this.

Our normative practices, therefore, as shown by the example of language, but also reflected in our judgements, are a part and parcel of our form of life, which includes the ways in which we engage with the world. They reflect the nature of our being-in-the-world. This suggests that certain types of engagement, or we could say certain sorts of judgement, are not optional, not completely contingent, but reflect ways in which we morally should (ought), to be in the world. We are, therefore, gesturing at something profound about the nature of our being as human beings of this type in the context of our worldly engagements as reflected by our patterns of language and thought.

Normativity is, on our view, to be found as an immanent, constitutive, and irreducible feature of our worldly engagements or patterned practices (Hughes 2011). However one wishes to pursue the philosophical arguments concerning the source (if there is such a thing) of normativity, its nature and existence (as manifest by our clinical and ethical judgements) entail that these judgements are inextricably linked with the broader nature of our being-in-the-world.

According to Luntley (2003) the key thing is that we should 'see the world aright'. He says this in an account of the philosophy of thought and language. However, his words are entirely apposite to the discussion of clinical and ethical judgements.

The conditions for judgement consist not in a body of theoretical knowledge, possession of which grants the subject with the capacity for using language, it consists in the subject seeing the world aright (Luntley 2003 p. 152).

By 'seeing the world aright' Luntley implies that the person must be 'an active subject, an agent with an attitude to the world' (*ibid.*). He goes on to say that the way language-users show they see things aright 'will be in their practice, their going on right', their having a certain attitude towards the world (*ibid.* p. 154). He says: 'Their correctness consists in their taking the right attitude to things, of setting their face to the world in the appropriate way' (*ibid.* p. 154).

One aspect that he wishes to emphasize is that these patterns of practice, with their inherent normativity, must entail more than a simple technique. The notion of engagement with the world points towards something more creative. This sort of creativity is an inherent feature of what it means to be a language-user, what it means, that is, to have meaning.

So we are not talking about simple procedures or techniques, because we are not disconnected atoms in the world. Our nature is to Be-with. This is fundamental. It also takes us back to the idea of good judgement generally, where this can now be conceived as seeing the world aright. So good clinical judgement fits into a pattern of practice that is constituted by taking the right attitude to things on the basis of experience, whether this is in the clinic, the classroom or the world.

A Practice is not an Algorithm

From what has already been said, therefore, it should be obvious that to be engaged in a normative practice is not simply to participate in a pathway of functional procedures. To make clinical and ethical judgements is to engage with others in ways that cannot be set down precisely. When we acquire practices in medical school, therefore, we cannot simply be learning algorithms. This is not to say that many clinical judgements cannot be described algorithmically, but it is to suggest that no algorithm can in the end completely depict all of the possibilities.

Our understanding of normativity as something immanent, constitutive and irreducible stands against the belief that the world itself and everything that it entails could be accurately specified and predicted. Normativity emerges inherently in the context of practice in particular circumstances, but it cannot then be reduced to any particular circumstances or any particular causes. The normativity that characterizes these sorts of practice cannot itself be given a normative construal. Instead, what is at stake is, to use Luntley's expression, that we should see the world aright, that we should see how to proceed, how to act, in particular circumstances. But this means having a broad view of the world. To bring us back to clinical practice, we have to see how one thing connects with another and how the whole makes sense. As Wittgenstein said: 'We do not learn the practice of making empirical judgements by learning rules: we are taught *judgements* and their connection with other judgements. *A totality* of judgements is made plausible to us' (Wittgenstein 1969 §140).

Hence, in medical school, although we shall learn algorithms, our judgements will in the end have to depend on more than algorithms. They will have to depend on our engagements with specific, particular circumstances and contexts (in the hospital, and also in the world) in which we must (where this reflects the normative constraint) see how we should act, partly by seeing the whole.

Tacit Knowledge and Judgement

Lying behind the idea that the world cannot be described algorithmically, is the notion of tacit knowledge. This suggests that there are things we cannot say but which do, nonetheless, inform our engagement with the world and our judgements about it. This tacit knowledge can be seen in the ways in which we deal practically with the world irrespective of theoretical understandings. The point may be put by saying that we cannot articulate the background framework according to which we make the interpretations that culminate in clinical or ethical judgements. It is tacit knowledge (Polanyi 1958). Of course we can articulate a background, but what is the further background according to which we understand this background? There must be something that acts as a given, which shows itself in our engagements with the world. Thornton, on the basis of Wittgensteinian arguments, puts it thus: 'Even when a form of judgement can be codified as the application of a principle or rule, the application of the rule still depends on an element of uncodified skill' (Thornton 2007 p. 222).

Clinical judgements are clearly based on codes and rules, but the interpretation that moves us from a symptom to a syndrome to a decision about treatment involves skills based on experience. Part of the relevant experience is our straightforward awareness of other people. At some point, this is based simply on our mode of being-in-the-world. And our Being-with also suggests something ethical. Given how we are in-the-world, we *ought* to behave in one way rather than in another. But this background (ethical) framework, the justification of which becomes at some point ineffable, is part of the normative element of clinical judgement. It is also a reflection of good judgement generally or of seeing the world aright.

Experience and Judgement

There are things that have to be presumed, they are tacit, for learning even to take place. Although facts can be taught, what must also be acquired to make clinical judgements is experience of the right sort. Judgement requires experience, which is another way to point towards engagement with the world. In a sense, this is inevitable. It is the 'pre-understanding' of Gadamer (1960). But the right sort of experience does not necessarily include exposure to lectures in medical ethics. Exposure to the humanities, to literature, art and music, may be more relevant. This is not to argue that philosophical skills will be irrelevant – far from it – although a certain detached analytic stance may not always be useful. No, the point is (again) that the clinician needs to have the right engagement with the world: he or she needs to see the world aright in order to make the correct judgements. These have to be made against the background of worldly encounters that constitute good judgement generally. Exposure to the humanities, therefore, is just a way of encouraging a broad understanding of the world.

Honing of the relevant human capacities will not be a matter of learning theories, principles or definitions. The key thing will be how we are able to engage with the world as human beings of this sort. We do not exclude the possibility that lectures in medical ethics might help. But the requisite understanding is much broader. Thus, as Wittgenstein says:

> What determines our judgement, our concepts and reactions, is not what *one* man is doing *now*, an individual action, but the whole hurly-burly of human actions, the background against which we see any action (Wittgenstein 1981 § 567).

Conclusion

Clinical encounters, which are particular, contextualized and inherently ethical, are made on the basis of our human encounters. We crudely characterized the acquisition of ethical know-how, the sort required for clinical judgements, as either being through osmosis, or as being didactically taught. We acknowledged the possibility, which may be increasingly normal, that ethical judgements are identified and discussed in the context of particular clinical judgements. This edges us towards the requisite simultaneity if clinical judgements are, at one and the same time, ethical judgements. But it does not take us all the way.

For, what is really required is a direct engagement with the clinical-as-ethical. To some extent, osmosis would do, if this does away with the gap in our thinking about clinical judgement: the gap that emerges between the clinical and the ethical. We need the right experience of the world. Our interpretations of this experience, however, rely on the unspoken background to the patterns of practice that we establish. This background, the hurly-burly of the world, against which our judgements are made, is broad. Ethics teaching is certainly *not* by the by. It gives us a language with which to articulate and understand this background. But nor is ethics the be-all and end-all. The crucial thing is the human encounter with the world, the nature of our Being-with that should characterize our Being-in-the-world.

It is in this worldly context that our patterns of practice can be seen to involve normativity. But this is not something that is added to the practices; it is immanent in and constitutive of these practices and is, moreover, irreducible. It is part of what it is for us to inhabit the forms of life that we do. From this perspective, therefore, our (inherently ethical) clinical judgements assume an importance that is distinct from the clinic and from the lecture theatre. Our clinical judgements are a means by which we engage with the world of 'Others'. We can learn about this by osmosis and from books. But in the end the rightness or wrongness of our judgements will depend on what we do in the particular circumstances of the case in a specific context against a normatively constrained background constituted by our human concerns.

Notes

Introduction

[1] One interesting but ham-fisted attempt at engagement with a Jehovah's Witness (JW) can be seen in Savulescu J. and Momeyer R. 'Should informed consent be based on rational beliefs?' in: *Journal of Medical Ethics*, vol. 23, 1997. For the purposes of their article, Savulescu and Momeyer are willing to accept the existence of the Christian God, but argue that it is the doctor's duty to attempt to persuade the JW, solely on the basis of scriptural interpretation, to abandon their blood-consumption beliefs as 'irrational'.

Chapter 1

[1] This chapter is based on two earlier publications of mine: Campbell and Willis (2006) and Campbell (2009). The reader is referred to these works for a fuller account of some of the arguments briefly outlined here.

[2] A full account of these exploitative factors will be found in Chapter Three of Campbell (2009).

[3] Some writers – e.g. Sykora (2010) – have argued that all such transactions involve *some* kind of reciprocity. While my gift may not gain me obvious commercial advantage, it may have other benefits such as improved social status or the warm glow of satisfaction from doing good. This may be true in some senses, but the argument is circular. Starting from the assumption that all deliberate actions will be motivated by something, it 'proves' that there is no purely altruistic gift. The point, however, is that some of the ends of our actions have a higher moral value than others. The motivation to create a caring society may be partly self-serving, but in essence it stems from a commitment to the welfare of all, even if there is no specific advantage to me in ensuring this.

Chapter 2

[1] 'A norm to a certain extent represents the objective side of the good life, and the wish for a good life represents the subjective side of ethical life' (Ricœur 2002 p. 282). For the sake of clarity in the bibliography, all publication dates refer to the English translations of Ricœur's works. But it should be kept in mind that the

translations were not published in chronological order to the original French and that some translations appeared long after Ricœur's death.

[2] For the history of *phronèsis* in Ricœur, see Fiasse 2008 pp. 349–360.

[3] For instance, no references to Ricœur are made in Beauchamp and Childress 2009; Kuhse and Singer 2009; May 2002; Sugarman and Sulmasy 2001.

[4] On the recent development of narrative medicine, see Dion-Labrie and Doucet 2011.

[5] For recent articles on the specific use of Ricœur's narrative identity, see Sitvast, Abma *et al.* 2008 pp. 268–279; Taiëb, Revah-Lévy *et al.* 2008 pp. 990–1000. On the use of Ricœur in medicine, see Qualtere-Burcher 2009; Dion-Labrie and Doucet 2011. For anthologies that briefly mention Ricœur, see Rehmann-Sutter and Düwell (eds.) 2006, ch. 23 by H. Haker, pp. 353–376; Khushf (ed.) 2004, the section by E. D. Pellegrino, p. 186.

[6] See endnote 5.

[7] For the role of promises in therapeutic relationships with drug addicts, in the light of Ricœur's philosophy, see Taiëb, Reyre, *et al.* 2010 pp. 21–34.

[8] Ricœur 2001 p. 116. This sentence gathers the ideas present in Article 7 of the French Deontological Code of medicine. See Ricœur 1996 pp. 63–64.

[9] 'Our responsibility grows as our power increases which in turn begets a supplementary fragility' (Ricœur 1993 p. 8).

[10] On the contrast between precepts and norms, see Ricœur 2007f p. 203.

Chapter 3

[1] Among those who have noticed that this may be valuable, see Hamrick (1974), Jacobson (2006) and Annas (2008). I also thank Erik Malmqvist for having pointed at this, in a personal communication.

[2] Hubert Dreyfus (2009) is an exception, though his study uses Merleau-Ponty in order to examine learning without brain representation.

[3] MacIntyre's and Pellegrino's account also differ from each other (see Pellegrino 2001). Since my aim is to show how practice and virtues can be conceptualized together, I shall not enter the discussion of how they differ. Furthermore, I will use to the common umbrella term of virtue ethics in this chapter even if some argue that virtue ethics is too loose a concept that only confuses discussions (Nussbaum 1999).

[4] MacIntyre's description of internal 'goods' has been criticized. For example, he states that internal 'goods' are internal in two senses: they can only be specified in terms of the practice at stake and they can only be identified by someone with experience of that practice. The latter idea has been criticized and it has been argued that the opposite may just as well be the case: when deeply engaged in a certain practice the subject may be biased in her or his understanding of that practice (see Thomasma 2000 p. 79).

[5] As put by Pellegrino again: 'What is "medically good" simply on grounds of physiological effectiveness may not be good,' if it violates higher levels of good, like the patient's good as he perceives that good' (Pellegrino 2001 p. 569).

[6] Dreyfus and Dreyfus (2004) note that most accounts of ethical competence see the moral subject as a competent actor who deliberates on alternative maxims and actions. This, they suggest, is because of the common philosophical mistake to read the structure of deliberation back into the skillful coping at stake when someone who has learnt to act ethically acts in a familiar but ethically complex situation. The mistake lay in not being able to discern the difference between (i) the deliberation involved when a moral subject who has learnt to act ethically, faces a problematic but familiar situation and (ii) that of her facing a novel one where she needs to fall back on abstract principles. They also give a reason why philosophers and ethicists have focused so much on reflective deliberation. Because of the tacit nature of ethical know-how, we are not aware of how much we rely on it in our everyday activities and this lack has fed into philosophical analyses. These have focused on what we are aware of, i.e. the less frequent processes of ethical reflective deliberation.

[7] Now, some may see the doctor's response as justified on the grounds of not unduly alarming the patient. Arguably, however, not responding – and not discussing the patient's worry – will not help the patient Ilych in coping with the situation. In other words, whereas warnings of danger can be unnecessary, the story of Ilych highlights the need for a more tuned-in interaction between doctor and patient.

[8] Skill models differ in their emphasis on the intellectual content of virtue as skill and on the importance attributed to the idea that subjects, having learnt a certain virtue, should be able to give an account of how they act or pinpoint the underlying principles for why they act as they do. This echoes the difference in views between Aristotle and Plato/Socrates on whether skills can be gained through experiences even if the subject does not acquire a thorough understanding of certain underlying principles of relevance for the practice. For excellent discussions of this, see Stichter 2007.

[9] Please note that, however, that which becomes incorporated will not be fully transparent and that the 'to-from' structure is not as clear-cut as the description above may lead us to assume. As discussed elsewhere (Malmqvist and Zeiler 2010), the transparency of the incorporated object can preferably be seen as an extension of the transparency of the lived body, and even if my bodily mode of being most often is pre-reflective and even if I do not attend to my own body in everyday activities, this transparency is never total. I will be pre-reflectively aware of my body *as* mine. There are nuances to be explored in relation to this 'to-from' structure. What if the stick breaks in the course of blind man's activity of seeing the world from it? What if the stick gets stuck in between two stones in the pavement when the man is out walking, which makes him unable to continue his walk as seamlessly as before? In such scenarios, the man will need to attend *to* the stick as an object of attention but he will need to do so *in his very activity of seeing the world from it.* Importantly, in the cases above, the stick does not stand forth as an object equal to other objects and the man will not attend *to* his stick in the same way as he previously, while it was incorporated, attended *from* it *to* other things. For discussion of this and other problems with this 'to-from' structure, see Zeiler 2012.

[10] One more clarification is needed. Consider the character Dr. House in the US hospital-TV program. This character is brilliant in the difficult task of giving correct diagnosis and treatment to patients' with rare conditions (and reluctantly admired); he is also very rude and insensitive to worries and anxieties on the part of his patients and colleagues. Whereas patients may prefer a competent but insensitive doctor instead of a nice but much less competent one, this way of putting it is to miss the point of this reasoning. The idea is not that scientific adequacy should be down-played, but that certain virtues-as-skills should be upgraded.

Chapter 5

[1] See *Palliative care in the European Union.* Downloaded on April 4 2011 at http://tinyurl.com/6ogtz5.

Chapter 7

[1] All the legal details of the case have been masterfully summarized (in English) and discussed in Griffiths 1995.

[2] Number supplied in personal correspondence with Ron Berghmans.

[3] The *Chabot* case is similar to the 1998 case of *Brongersma*, where PAS was granted to an elderly patient who claimed to be 'tired of life'. See Huxtable and Moller 2007. My arguments for refusing PAS to Mrs. Bosscher would apply even more strongly here.

[4] For reasons I have discussed elsewhere (Cowley 2006), I do not believe a suicide can be rational or irrational. This is because the concept of rationality makes an essential reference to the future, and suicide removes the future.

[5] Warnock and MacDonald (p. 25) give the example of Philip Graham, who killed himself during a lucid, non-depressed state because he feared the consequences for himself and his family of his next depressive episode. I would take this as an example similar to the suffering anticipated by a patient with a progressive somatic condition such as motor neurone disease, and as such I, for one, would not object to a Dutch doctor assisting such a person's suicide.

[6] However, I can accept the therapeutic value of reifying the depression in order to allow the patient to fight 'it' better.

[7] In the example, Robin was considered to be sufficiently at risk that he was sectioned under the Mental Health Act for a period of six months, during which time he co-operated in taking his medication and gradually lost his desire to kill himself. The question then is whether Mrs. Bosscher should have been treated in the same way, as the Dutch Supreme Court seemed to advocate.

[8] This conception of joint decision-making under a 'deliberative' and/or 'relational' model of autonomy is brought out by Widdershoven (2002), and represents an important challenge to the prevailing 'liberal' view of autonomy as

merely the absence of obstacles. In the case of a Dutch cancer patient, she might well discuss the possibility of euthanasia with friends and family, but only come to make up her mind during extended discussions with her doctor.

[9] It's true that Mrs. Bosscher might be a Christian, and might want not annihilation but to join her sons in the next world. If so, the situation would be complicated by the general Christian prohibition against suicide. There would then be a further dilemma for the doctor about whether to engage Mrs. Bosscher in a theological argument.

[10] In 2009, the UK Director of Public Prosecutions issued an interim policy describing the conditions for the state to refrain from prosecuting the assistance of suicide. See: http://www.cps.gov.uk/news/press_releases/144_09/ [accessed June 2011].

[11] My thanks to Guy Widdershoven, David Levy, Christopher Hamilton, and Cliona McGovern for comments on earlier drafts.
This book went to press before I could make use of a fascinating interview with Dr. Chabot in Thomasma D. *et al.* (1998) *Asking to Die: Inside the Dutch Debate about Euthanasia*, London: Kluwer. pp. 373–385.

Chapter 8

[1] It should be clear that these forms of attention to a person are not forms of *treatment*, but an ethical practice of medicine. They are therefore unrelated to injunctions to treat the whole person, not her body.

[2] Critiques of consequentialism that reach similar conclusions include Maclean 1993; Oderberg 2000; Smart and Williams 1973.

[3] As it were, the formal must become material. It adds nothing to define courage as a virtue oriented toward a worthy goal, because this is still formal rather than material. It lacks content.

[4] Cf. Parfit 1984, Appendix I for three groupings of ideas for assessing the quality of lives, viz. Hedonistic, Desire-Fulfillment and Objective List. These correspond roughly to actual pleasure experienced; satisfaction of one's goals or interests; and realization of a list of positive life properties.

[5] Kant (1785) *Groundwork of the Metaphysics of Morals*; e.g. Burgess 1972.

[6] The intended contrast is between practical and theoretical. Domains with theoretical and applied aspects, like mathematics, illustrate the difference. Applied mathematics uses specific techniques to solve problems, e.g. differential analysis. There is no analog to 'problems' or 'techniques' in theoretical mathematics. Ordinarily, no one is surprised when an applied mathematical problem is solved; not so for a theoretical discovery.

[7] The term 'consequentialism' was invented by Anscombe 1958. She applied the term to ethical theories that denied for moral responsibility a distinction between intended and foreseen consequences. This aspect of the definition re-appears in the section 'Two Arguments'.

[8] For the deontologist, questions of moral responsibility will begin with, 'what was the intention of this action?' with less regard to the action's actual consequences.

[9] Another way to conceive justice – viz. as the outcome of just or legitimate processes – yields different, weaker objections.

[10] For an early variant of motive consequentialism, see Adams 1976.

[11] A refinement in which what are valued are states of affairs, in which autonomous preferences and desires are satisfied by autonomous actions of those whose preferences and desires they are, is not promising as a rejoinder. For it requires selecting actions among whose outcomes are determinations of the autonomous actions of others, something I have argued is not possible.

Chapter 9

[1] Religion Versus Medicine blog (2010) 'Christian Medical fellowship and demonic possession of the mentally disordered', 28 May 2010 <http://religionversusmedicine.blogspot.com/2010/05/christian-medical-fellowship-and.html> [accessed March 2011]

[2] See University of Chicago Medical Center (2007) 'Psychiatrists: Least Religious But Most Interested In Patients' Religion'. http://www.sciencedaily.com/releases/2007/12/071210163123.htm [accessed March 2011]

Chapter 10

[1] Both cases are assumed to take place under the British state-funded National Healthcare System.

[2] In the discussion we assume patient autonomy in medical decision-making. Given the length of this paper this is an assumption we cannot defend here, but it has been well discussed in the general literature.

[3] An exception to this is the lively debate on the problem of 'moral luck' but we take this to be a separate issue, and even within this issue there is little discussion of the concept of 'luck' as such. The same seems to be true of discussions of epistemic luck which are significant but tangential to the topic of luck as such.

[4] This of course presumes belief in free will of some kind.

[5] We are adopting an account of luck which emphasizes on responsibility rather than deserting, a defense of which can be found in Zimmerman (1993 pp. 219–234) and Cohen (1989 p. 916).

[6] They are also prominent in the debate that has taken place about the extent to which there is a just requirement to treat patients who are, to some extent, implicated in the occurrence of their disease – a debate in which Dworkin's distinction between brute and option luck (Dworkin 2000) plays a significant role. We have chosen not to discuss the issue of 'responsibility for illness' in this paper because it is an issue which requires lengthy treatment which might distract from our main thesis. In addition, the Dworkonian distinction features extensively in debate on this topic and we think this distinction is misleading. In our view 'option luck' is

better thought of as 'risk' and consequently best judged by the moral standards appropriate to risk-taking.

7 Procedural fairness, as used here, is fairness in the process by which prioritization takes place. So in this case a procedurally fair policy would be one which was democratic, transparent etc. The NHS may not be a democratic institution but in such matters it carries out the mandate of an elected government and its procedures for priority setting are governed by NICE guidelines and open to challenge in the courts (as in the Herceptin case).

Chapter 11

1 I would like to thank Lindsay Stirton, Jurgen De Wispelaere, Joanna Shapland, Aurora Plomer and the redliners.

2 This is a common challenge made to the Millian harm principle. Mill considers harm to be a prejudicial effect on another's interests (Mill 1985 p. 141) while the relevant others are 'our fellow creatures' (Mill 1985 p. 71). There is some academic work exploring the harm arising from genetic decision-making: Lucassen and Parker (2004); and who the others are: Wilkinson (2010a).

3 See Wilkinson (2010a), where I argued that while it is possible to advise individuals which others might be relevant, only that individual decision maker can really know who is important.

4 In the HIV example, you may be responsible for your partner's risk. In that respect there is a difference between these two scenarios, which might be sufficient to justify distinct regulatory regimes. But what if we change HIV to swine flu? Knowing that your partner has swine flu is not something you are necessarily responsible for. It also tells you something about your risk of contracting the illness. Is there really a sufficient difference between these two to justify wholly different regimes?

5 See Diver and Maslow Cohen (2001), Hellman (2003), Wilkinson (2010b) for further explorations of the difficulties of defining genetic discrimination.

6 There is a real question about whether it is appropriate to single out genetic information for a specific regulatory regime. Insurance companies have always based their assessments of risk on family medical history. In many cases, the family history will provide them with more than enough information. But, banning the use of family history information would fundamentally undermine the concept of insurance to the extent that a private insurance industry may no longer be viable.

7 See Lowe, Z. (2010) 'Paul Hastings fights genetic discrimination claims under new law' in: the blog *American Law Daily*, http://amlawdaily.typepad.com/amlawdaily/2010/05/genetic-discrimination.html (accessed June 2010).

8 For a discussion of UK employment concerns, see Godard *et al.* (2003).

9 The moratorium has been in place since 1999, and has been renewed every few years. The next review, and renewal, is expected in 2017.

10 This is an issue for another paper, but it is worth considering that this problem may be more acute for people with a chronic illness which makes them look well,

or even for chronically ill people who have made an effort to look well. In this situation the social perception will be that nothing is wrong with them;that they are faking. This could be extremely damaging.

Chapter 12

[1] See also e.g. *Portsmouth* 2006. Bridgeman (2010) refers to there being at least 11 hearings.

[2] I will use 'ethics' and 'morals' interchangeably in this chapter.

[3] Unlike with formal rationality, here the concern is with whether law can guide action. Contradictory law obviously cannot do so and neither can unclear nor frequently fluctuating legal rules – so (unlike formal rationality) instrumental rationality requires attention to any tensions between doctrines.

[4] It is notable that, although Fuller did not attribute his eight principles to any secure point of reference (cf. Morrison (1997, p. 389), he edited the volume containing Beale's thesis prior to the publication of *The Morality of Law.*

[5] I am alert to the controversy that surrounds appeals to rationality and logic, particularly in light of feminist critiques (Falmagne and Hass 2002). Although it will surely not suffice, the best I can do is wager that none of us would want (or so label) a system of law which issues flatly contradictory instructions. From this most simple principle has evolved much of the framework for judging 'law' as defended here.

[6] Grateful thanks to the Wellcome Trust, for providing research funding support in the period in which this paper was written.

Chapter 13

[1] In September 2003, Dr. Michael Neary, a consultant obstetrician and gynaecologist, was struck off the medical register following a decision by the Fitness to Practice Committee of the Irish Medical Council. In 1998, two midwives working in the maternity unit in Neary's hospital reported that Neary was carrying out an unusual number of caesarean hysterectomies, also called peripartum hysterectomies. A peripartum hysterectomy is an emergency procedure that could be carried out if a woman, after giving birth, had severe uterine bleeding which could not be stopped by any other measure. Typically, there is a higher risk of needing a peripartum hysterectomy after a caesarean delivery but it remains a rare procedure. When the official Inquiry into Neary's practices released its findings, it stated that during the 1980s and 1990s the rate of peripartum hysterectomy at Lourdes Hospital far exceeded the worst figures at the three Dublin Maternity hospitals, even though rates of delivery in each of the Dublin hospitals were three times higher (see p. 95 of the Inquiry).

[2] Most of the cases involving Dr Neary were 'statute barred' as plaintiffs have three years from the time of knowledge of an alleged negligence to bring proceedings. Instead, an Inquiry was established and a redress scheme was introduced for

the victims. 119 women were awarded sums between €60,000 and €380,000 each and the total cost of the scheme came to €20.6 million. See Culliton G, 'Redress scheme cost €20.6 million', *Irish Medical Times*19 May 2011.

[3] Dr Bernard Stuart, Dr John Murphy and Prof Walter Prendiville.

[4] See also, *O'Laoire v. The Medical Council* (1995) (HC).

[5] 'An order of certiorari' means to bring a decision of a lower court or tribunal to a higher court to review the decision and quash it if necessary.

[6] Bolam v Friern Hospital Management Committee [1957] 1 WLR 582.

[7] EMI Records (Ireland) Ltd v UPC Communications Ireland Ltd [2011] ECC 8 215.

[8] The three professions were a) Rugby Union b) Medicine and c) Physiotherapy.

[9] Sky Sports paid £20 million for the rights for three years. Clubs earn a portion of this money and the further up the championship they progress, the more money they earn in addition to prize money and advertising revenue.

[10] Brennan was also the physiotherapist for the English rugby team. He was at the pinnacle of his career, with high profiles jobs at club and international level, so it is hard to believe that he is the man who brought his profession into such disrepute.

[11] In the UK, under the Health Professions Order 2001, the independent Health Professions Council was established. They regulate fifteen autonomous professions including physiotherapists.

[12] Health Professions Council, Fitness to Practice Section, Conduct and Competence Committee Hearing on Stephen Brennan, 18 May 2011.

[13] Under the Health Professions Order 2001, a person has 28 days to appeal the outcome of the Competence and Conduct Committee to the courts.

[14] See R. (on the application of Howlett) v Health Professions Council [2009] EWHC 3617 (Admin).

[15] *Bolton v Law Society* [1994] 1 WLR 512, 519.

[16] Note, this is not what happened in *Prendiville,* where the courts quashed the findings and did not remit the matter back to the Medical Council. For the Brennan remittal, see *Brennan* para 65.

[17] Health Professions Council, Fitness to Practice Section, Conduct and Competence Committee Hearing on Stephen Brennan, 18 May 2011.

[18] An intimate examination in these circumstances refers to a digital examination of the patient's rectum or vagina (or both) while the patient is under anesthesia. These examinations are carried out because, usually, the patient has presented with atypical symptoms and this is an opportunity for the student doctor to learn, for example, what a cancerous tumor of the prostrate gland feels like. Such a symptom would not usually be present in any of the bodies that medical students use for anatomy dissection. However, in some medical schools, abdominal simulators like the 'Tummy Dummy' are used to teach students about how to perform vaginal and rectal examinations. While it is not documented anywhere, it has been known for medical students to be instructed to perform intimate examinations on anaesthetized patients who have presented in the theatre with, perhaps, appendicitis or even tonsillitis. One would sincerely hope that this no longer happens.

[19] Schloendorff v Society of NY Hospital, 105 NE 92 (NY 1914).

Chapter 14

[1] Available online at http://www.pfli.org/main.php?pfli = modelpharmacistcc [accessed February 2011]

[2] Physicians who are not asked to act against their conscience may value their moral integrity no less than objecting physicians, but the former do not face the same threats to their moral integrity as physicians who are asked to act against their conscience.

[3] Generally, considerable deference should be given to the beliefs of objectors. However, there are some exceptions. Doctors should not expect to be accommodated if their conscience-based refusals are undoubtedly incompatible with the goals of medicine. For example, suppose Mathias believes that patients' pain and suffering should not be alleviated because they are God's punishment for evil deeds. Mathias should not become a general practitioner.

[4] Physicians with a conscience-based objection to performing abortions might deny that pregnancy is a *medical* condition and deny that abortion is a *medical* procedure. However it is not up to objectors to set the boundaries of acceptable professional practice. Although efforts can and should be made to accommodate individual physicians who believe that pregnancy is not a medical condition and abortion is not a medical procedure, they do not have the authority to determine for the medical profession and patients what is and is not a 'medical procedure' and which needs are and are not 'medical needs'.

[5] Levonorgestrel based EC (Plan B) is effective for up to 3 days after unprotected intercourse. Ulipristal acetate based EC (ellaOne in European Union countries and ella in the United States) is effective up to 5 days after unprotected intercourse.

[6] See for example Abbott 2005, Foster *et al.* 2004 and Merchant *et al.* 2007.

[7] The constraint against blocking patient access applies only to legal and clinically suitable medical goods and services. It does not apply to 'futile' or 'medically inappropriate' treatment.

[8] This description of the case is based on the accounts provided in a California Supreme Court decision, *North Coast Women's Care Medical Group, Inc. v. San Diego County Superior Court* (189 P 3d 959 [Cal. 2008]); Moran 2005 and Buchanan 2005.

[9] At the time when Dr. Brody told Ms. Benitez that she would not provide IUI, the Unruh Civil Rights Act did not explicitly prohibit discrimination on the basis of sexual orientation. However, courts had interpreted the statute to include such a prohibition. An amendment enacted in 2005 expressly prohibits discrimination on the basis of sexual orientation and marital status (Ca. Stats. 2005 ch. 420 § 2.). Among the legal questions raised by the case is whether the protection of religious liberty in federal and state law exempts individuals from the anti-discrimination provisions of the Unruh Civil Rights Act. The California Supreme Court in 2008 held that there is no such exemption (189 P 3d 959 [Cal. 2008]).

Bibliography

Abbott, J. (2005) 'Emergency contraception: what should our patients expect?' *Annals of Emergency Medicine* 46(2): 111–13.

Adams, J. and Brownsword, R. (1995) *Key Issues in Contract.* London: Butterworths.

Adams, R. M. (1976) 'Motive utilitarianism'. *The Journal of Philosophy* 73(14): 467–481.

Agich, G. (1993) *Autonomy and Long-Term Care.* New York/Oxford: Oxford University Press.

—. (2003) *Dependence and Autonomy in Old Age.* Cambridge: Cambridge University Press.

—. (2007) 'Autonomy as a problem for clinical ethics'. In: Nys, T., Denier, Y., and Vandevelde, A. (eds) *Autonomy and Paternalism.* Leuven/Paris/Dudley, MA: Peeters, pp. 71–91.

Ahmed, S. (2006) *Queer Phenomenology: Orientations, Objects, Others.* Durham/London: Duke University Press.

Ahmedzai, S. (1993) 'The medicalization of dying. A doctor's view'. In: Clark, D. (ed.) *The Future for Palliative Care.* Oxford: Oxford University Press.

Ahronheim, J., Moreno, J. and Zuckerman, C. (eds) (1994) *Ethics in Clinical Practice.* Boston/New York/Toronto/London: Little, Brown and Company.

Andrews, L. B. (1986) 'My body, my property'. *Hastings Center Report* 16(5): 28–38.

Andrews, L. B. and Nelkin, D. (2001) *Body Bazaar: The Market for Human Tissue in the Biotechnology Age.* New York: Crown Publishers.

Annas, G. J. (1999) 'Genetic privacy: there ought to be a law'. *Texas Review of Law and Politics* 4(2): 9–16.

Annas, J. (2004) 'Being virtuous and doing the right thing'. *Proceedings and Addresses of the American Philosophical Association* 78(2): 61–75.

—. (2008) 'The phenomenology of virtue'. *Phenomenology and the Cognitive Science* 7: 21–34.

Anonymous. (2005) 'Moralists at the pharmacy'. *New York Times,* 3 April 2005, p. 12.

Anscombe, G. E. M. (1958) 'Modern moral philosophy'. *Philosophy* 33(124): 1–19.

Archard, D. (2002) 'Selling yourself: Titmuss's argument against a market in blood'. *Journal of Ethics* 6(11): 87–103.

Ashcroft, R. (2007) 'Should genetic information be disclosed to insurers? No'. *British Medical Journal* 334: 1197.

Athanassoulis, N. (2005) *Morality, Moral Luck and Responsibility.* Basingstoke: Palgrave.

Athanassoulis, N. and Ross, A. (2010) 'A virtue ethical account of making decisions about risk'. *Journal of Risk Research* 13(2): 217–230.

—. (2011) 'Risk ad virtue ethics'. In: Roeser, S. (ed.) *Handbook of Risk Theory.* New York: Springer.

Audi, R. (2010) 'Moral perception and moral knowledge'. *Aristotelian Society Supplementary Volume* 84(1): 79–97.

St. Augustine. (1982) *St. Augustine, the Literal Meaning of Genesis. vol. 1,* Ancient Christian Writers, vol. 41. Taylor (tr.) New York: Paulist Press.

Badham, P. (2005) 'Welcome to the Christian deathbed'. *Church Times* 7440, 14 October 2005.

Beale, J. H. (1935) 'The nature of law'. In: Fuller, L. L. (ed.) *The Problems of Jurisprudence: A Selection of Readings Supplemented by Comments Prepared by the Editor* (temporary edn). Brooklyn, NY: The Foundation Press, pp. 346–355.

Beauchamp, T. L. and Childress, J. F. (2009) *Principles of Biomedical Ethics,* 6th ed. New York/Oxford: Oxford University Press.

de Beauvoir, S. (2003/1949) *The Second Sex.* New York: Alfred A. Knopf.

Bell, D. and Bennett, B. (2001) 'Genetic secrets and the family'. *Medical Law Review* 9: 130–161.

Benner, P. (1997) 'A dialogue between virtue ethics and care ethics'. *Theoretical Medicine* 18: 47–61.

Berghmans, R. (1998) 'Commentary on "suicide, euthanasia and the psychiatrist"'. *Philosophy, Psychiatry & Psychology* 5(2): 131–135.

Berlin, I. (1958) *Two Concepts of Liberty.* Oxford: Clarendon Press.

Beyleveld, D. and Brownsword, R. (2001) *Human Dignity in Bioethics and Biolaw.* Oxford: Oxford University Press.

—. (1994) *Law as a Moral Judgment.* Sheffield: Sheffield Academic Press.

Biswas, B. (1993) 'The medicalization of dying. A nurse's view'. In: Clark, D. (ed.) *The Future for Palliative Care.* Oxford: Oxford University Press.

Bolsin, S., Faunce, T. and Oakley, J. (2005) 'Practical virtue ethics: healthcare whistleblowing and portable digital technology'. *Journal of Medical Ethics* 31(10): 612–618.

Bradshaw, A. (1996) 'The spiritual dimension of hospice. The secularization of an ideal'. *Social Science and Medicine* 43: 409–419.

Bridgeman, J. (2010) 'Editorial: critically ill children and best interests'. *Clinical Ethics* 5: 184–187.

Bristol Royal Infirmary Inquiry. (2000) *Interim Report of the Bristol Royal Infirmary Inquiry.* London: Central Office of Information.

Brock, D. (2008) 'Conscientious refusal by physicians and pharmacists: who is obligated to do what, and why?' *Theoretical Medicine and Bioethics* 29: 187–200.

Brody, H. (2002) *Stories of Sickness.* Oxford. Oxford University Press.

Brooke, J. H. (1991) *Science and Religion: Some Historical Perspectives.* Cambridge: Cambridge University Press.

Brownsword, R. (1993) 'Towards a rational law of contract'. In: Wilhelmsson, T. (ed.) *Perspectives of Critical Contract Law.* Aldershot: Dartmouth, pp. 241–272.

—. (1996) "Good faith in contracts' revisited'. *Current Legal Problems* 49: 111–157.

—. (1997) 'From co-operative contracting to a contract of co-operation'. In: Campbell, D. and Vincent-Jones, P. (eds) *Contract and Economic Organisation.* Aldershot: Dartmouth, pp. 14–39.

Buchanan, A. and Brock, D. (1989) *Deciding for Others.* Cambridge: Cambridge University Press.

Buchanan, W. (2005) 'Doctor and patient both say their liberty was violated'. *San Francisco Chronicle*, 29 July 2005, p. A1.

Buiting, H., *et al.* (2009) 'Reporting of euthanasia and physician-assisted suicide in the Netherlands: descriptive study'. *BMC Medical Ethics*. 10(18) [published on-line so no page numbers].

Burgess, A. (1972) *A Clockwork Orange*. Harmondsworth: Penguin.

Burgess, S. and Hawton, K. (1998) 'Suicide, euthanasia and the psychiatrist'. *Philosophy, Psychiatry & Psychology* 5(2): 113–126.

Campbell, A. V. (1984) *Moderated Love: A Theology of Professional Care*. London: SPCK.

—. (2009) *The Body in Bioethics*. London/New York: Cavendish.

Campbell, A., Gillett, G. and Jones, G. (2005) *Medical Ethics*, 4th ed. Melbourne/Oxford/New York: Oxford University Press.

Campbell, A. V. and Willis, M. (2006) 'They stole my baby's soul: narratives of embodiment and loss'. *Medical Humanities* 31(2): 101–104; reprinted in Rapport, F. and Wainwright, P. (eds) *The Self in Health and Illness*. Oxford: Radcliffe, pp. 123–130.

Cantor, J. and Baum, K. (2004) 'The limits of conscientious objection—may pharmacists refuse to fill prescriptions for emergency contraception?' *New England Journal of Medicine* 351(19): 2008–2012.

Carel, H. (2008) *Illness: The Cry of the Flesh*. Durham, NC: Acumen.

Casarett, D. J. (1999) 'Moral perception and the pursuit of medical philosophy'. *Theoretical Medicine and Bioethics* 20(2): 125–139.

CBCEW. (2010) Catholic Bishops'. Conference of England & Wales Dept. for Christian Responsibility & Citizenship, *A Practical Guide to The Spiritual Care of the Dying Person*. London: CTS.

Charo, R. (2005) 'The celestial fire of conscience—refusing to deliver medical care'. *New England Journal of Medicine* 352(24): 2471–2473.

Chervenak, F. and McCullough, L. B. (2008) 'The ethics of direct and indirect referral for termination of pregnancy'. *American Journal of Obstetrics and Gynecology* 199: 232.e1–232.e3.

Chief Medical Officer's Summit on Organ Retention. (2001) *Evidence Documentation*. London: Department of Health.

Clark, D. (1999) 'Total pain, disciplinary power and the body in the work of Cicely Saunders, 1958–1967'. *Social Science and Medicine* 49: 727–736.

—. (2000) 'Palliative care history. A ritual process?' *European Journal of Palliative Care* 7(2): 50–55.

—. (2001) 'Religion, medicine, and community in the early origins of St. Christopher's hospice'. *Journal of Palliative Medicine* 4(3): 353–360.

Clark, D., *et al.* (2002) 'Palliative care service developments in seven European countries'. In: Ten Have, H. and Clark, D. (eds) *The ethics of palliative care. European Perspectives*. Oxford: Oxford University Press, pp. 34–51.

Cohen, G. (1989) 'The currency of egalitarian justice'. *Ethics* 99: 906–944.

Cohen-Almagor, R. (2002) 'Should doctors suggest euthanasia to their patients? Reflections on Dutch perspectives'. *Theoretical Medicine* 23: 287–303.

Coldicott, Y., Pope, C. and Roberts, C. (2003) 'The ethics of intimate examinations—teaching tomorrow's doctors'. *British Medical Journal* 326: 97–99.

Council on Ethical and Judicial Affairs. (2010) *Code of Medical Ethics of the American Medical Association*. Chicago, IL: American Medical Association.

Cowley, C. (2006) 'Suicide is neither rational nor irrational'. *Ethical Theory and Moral Practice* 9(5): 495–504.

Cox, S. M. and McKellin, W. (1999) "There's this thing in our family': predictive testing and the construction of risk for Huntington's disease'. *Sociology of Health and Illness* 21(5): 622–646.

Craig, P. (1997) 'Formal and substantive conceptions of the rule of law: an analytical framework'. *Public Law* 1997: 467–487.

Culliton, G. (2011) 'Redress scheme cost •20.6 million'. *Irish Medical Times*, 19 May 2011.

Damasio, A. R. (1999) *The Feeling of What Happens: Body and Emotion in the Making of Consciousness.* New York: Harcourt Brace.

Davidson, L., Shaw, J., Welborn, S., Mahon, B., Sirota, M., Gilbo, P., McDermid, M., Fazio, J., Breetz, S. and Pelletier, J.-F. (2010) "I don't know how to find my way in the world': contributions of user-led research to transforming mental health practice'. *Psychiatry* 73(2): 101–113.

Dawkins, P. (1997) 'Is science a religion?' *The Humanist*, January/February 1997. Accessed March 2011, <http://www.thehumanist.org/humanist/articles/dawkins.html>.

Dennett, D. C. (1984) *Elbow Room.* Oxford: Clarendon Press.

Department of Health, Association of British Insurers. (2005) *Concordat and Moratorium on Genetics and Insurance.* Available from the Department of Health website: http://www.dh.gov.uk/ [accessed 25 November 2011].

Descartes, R. (1988) *Selected Philosophical Writings.* Cottingham, J., Stoothoff, R., and Murdoch, D. (trs.). Cambridge: Cambridge University Press.

Devlin, P. (1965) *The Enforcement of Morals.* Oxford: Oxford University Press.

Dion-Labrie, M. and Doucet, H. (2011) 'Médecine narrative et éthique narrative en Amérique du Nord: perspective historique et critique. À la recherche d'une médecine humaniste'. *Ethique & Santé* 8(2): 63–68.

Diver, C. S. and Maslow Cohen, J. (2001) 'Genophobia: what is wrong with genetic discrimination?' *University of Pennsylvania Law Review* 149(5): 1439–1482.

Doyal, L. (1990) 'Medical ethics and moral indeterminacy'. *Journal of Law and Society* 17(1): 1–16.

Doyle, D., *et al.* (1996) 'Introduction'. In: Doyle, D., *et al.* (eds) *The Oxford Textbook of Palliative Medicine.* Oxford: Oxford University Press, pp. 3–8.

Dreyfus, H. L. (2009) 'A Phenomenology of Skill Acquisition as the basis for a Merleau-Pontian Nonrepresentationalist Cognitive Science', unpublished manuscript, available at: http://www-personal.umich.edu/~lormand/phil/teach/mmm/readings/Dreyfus%20-%20NonRepresentationalist%20Cognitive%20Science.pdf [accessed April 2011]

Dreyfus, H. L. and Dreyfus, S. E. (2004) 'The ethical implications of the five-stage skill-acquisition model'. *Bulletin of Science, Technology and Society* 24(3): 251–264.

Dworkin, R. (1985) *A Matter of Principle.* Cambridge, MA: Harvard University Press.

—. (1993) *Life's Dominion.* London: Harper/Collins Publishers.

—. (2000) *Sovereign Virtue: The Theory and Practice of Equality.* Cambridge, MA: Harvard University Press.

Ehman, J. W., Ott, B. B., Short, T. H., Ciampa, R. C. and Hansen-Flaschen, J. (1999) 'Do patients want physicians to inquire about their spiritual or religious beliefs if they become gravely ill?' *Archives of Internal Medicine* 159: 1803–1806.

Erin, C. A. and Harris, J. (2003) 'An ethical market in human organs'. *Journal of Medical Ethics* 29: 137–138.

Falmagne, R. J. and Hass, M. (eds) (2002) *Representing Reason: Feminist Theory and Formal Logic.* Lanham, MD: Rowman and Littlefield.

Farmer, F. (1983) *Will There Really be a Morning?* Glasgow: William Collins Sons & Co.

Farr, A. D. (1983) 'Religious opposition to obstetric anaesthesia: a myth?' *Annals of Science* 409: 159–177.

Feinberg, J. (1986) *The Moral Limits of the Criminal Law, Vol. 3: Harm to Self.* Oxford/ New York: Oxford University Press

Ferngren, G. (ed.) (2002) *Science & Religion: A Historical Introduction.* Baltimore, MD: Johns Hopkins University Press.

—. (2009) (ed.) *Medicine and Health Care in Early Christianity.* Baltimore, MD: Johns Hopkins University Press.

Fiasse, G. (2008) 'La *phronèsis* dans l'éthique de Paul Ricœur'. In: Lories, D. and Rizzerio, L. (eds) *Le jugement pratique: Autour de la notion de phronèsis.* Paris: J. Vrin, pp. 349–360.

—. (2010) 'The golden rule and forgiveness'. In: Treanor, B. and Venema, H. I. (eds) *A Passion for the Possible. Thinking with Paul Ricœur.* New York: Fordham University Press, pp. 77–89.

Field, D. (1994) 'Palliative medicine and the medicalization of death'. *European Journal of Cancer Care* 3: 58–62.

Finnis, J. (1986) *Natural Law and Natural Rights.* Oxford: Clarendon Press.

Foster, D. G., *et al.* (2004) 'Knowledge of emergency contraception among women aged 18 to 44 in California'. *American Journal of Obstetrics and Gynecology* 191: 150–156.

Foucault, M. (1975) *The Birth of the Clinic: An Archaeology of Medical Perception.* Smith, A.M.S. (tr.). New York: Vintage Books.

Frey, B. B., Daaleman, T. P. and Peyton, V. (2005) 'Measuring a dimension of spirituality for health research: validity of the spirituality index of well-being'. *Research on Aging* 27(5): 556–577.

Fulford, K. W. M. (1989) *Moral Theory and Medical Practice.* Cambridge: Cambridge University Press.

—. (2004) 'Facts/values: ten principles of values based medicine'. In: Radden, J. (ed.) *The Philosophy of Psychiatry—A Companion.* Oxford: Oxford University Press, pp. 205–234.

Fuller, L. L. (1969) *The Morality of Law* (revised edition). New Haven, CT: Yale University Press.

Gadamer, H.-G. (1960). *Wahrheit und Methode.* Tübingen: Mohr. (Translated as *Truth and Method,* revised ed. (1989) Weinsheimer, J. and Marshall, D. G. (trs.). London/New York: Continuum.)

Gardiner, P. (2003) 'A virtue ethics approach to moral dilemmas in medicine'. *Journal of Medical Ethics* 29: 297–302.

General Medical Council. (2006) *Good Medical Practice* (updated 2009). London: GMC.

—. (2008) *Personal Beliefs and Medical Practice—Guidance for Doctors.* London: GMC.

—. (2010) *Treatment and Care Towards the End of Life: Good Practice in Decision Making.* London: GMC.

Gewirth, A. (1978) *Reason and Morality*. Chicago, IL: University of Chicago Press.
Godard, B., Raeburn, S., Pembrey, M., Bobrow, M., Farndon, P. and Aymé, S. (2003) 'Genetic information and testing in insurance and employment: technical, social and ethical issues'. *European Journal of Human Genetics* 11(Suppl 2): S123–S142.
Gormally, L. (1997) 'Medicine as a profession and the meaning of health as its goal'. *Briefing* 27: 14–19.
Gould, S. J. (1997) 'Nonoverlapping magisteria'. *Natural History* 106: 16–22.
Gracia, D. (2002) 'Palliative care and the historical background'. In: Ten Have, H. and Clark, D. (eds) *The Ethics of Palliative Care. European Perspectives*. Oxford: Oxford University Press, pp. 18–33.
Graham, G. (1990) 'Melancholic epistemology'. *Synthese* 82: 399–422.
Green, M. and Botkin, J. (2003) "Genetic exceptionalism' in medicine: clarifying the differences between genetic and nongenetic tests'. *Annals of Internal Medicine* 138: 571–575.
Griffiths, J. (1995) 'Suicide in the Netherlands: the Chabot case'. *The Modern Law Review* 58(2): 232–248.
Hamrick, S. (1974) 'Whitehead and Merleau-Ponty: some moral implications'. *Process Studies* 4(4): 235–251.
Harding Clark, M. (2006) *An Inquiry into Peripartum Hysterectomy at Our Lady of Lourdes Hospital, Drogheda*. Dublin: Irish Government Publication Office.
Harris, J. (2002) 'Law and regulation of retained organs: the ethical issues'. *Legal Studies* 22: 527–549.
—. (2003) 'Organ procurement: dead interests, living needs'. *Journal of Medical Ethics* 29: 130–134.
Hart, H. L. A. (1963) *Law, Liberty and Morality*. Oxford: Oxford University Press.
—. (1965) 'Review: Fuller, *The Morality of Law*'. *Harvard Law Review* 78: 1281–1296.
Heidegger, M. (1962/1927) *Being and Time*. Macquarrie, J. and Robinson, E. (trs.). Oxford: Basil Blackwell.
—. (1977) (1993/2011) *Basic writings: From Being and time (1927) to The task of thinking (1964)*. London/New York: Routledge.
—. (1987) (2001) *Zollikon Seminars: Protocols—Conversations—Letters*. Boss, M. (ed.) Mayr, F. and Askay, R. (trs.). Illinois: Northwestern University Press.
Hellman, D. (2003) 'What makes genetic discrimination exceptional?' *American Journal of Law and Medicine* 29: 77–116.
Hermsen, M., *et al.* (2001) 'Moral problems in palliative care journals'. *Palliative Medicine* 15(5): 425–431.
Herring, J. and Chau, P. L. (2007) 'My body, your body, our bodies'. *Medical Law Review* 15: 34–61.
Hodge, J. (1995) *Heidegger and Ethics*. London/New York: Routledge.
Holm, S. (2007) 'Should genetic information be disclosed to insurers? Yes'. *British Medical Journal* 334: 1198–1198.
Honoré, T. (1961) 'Ownership'. In: Guest, A. G. (ed.) *Oxford Essays in Jurisprudence: A Collaborative Work*. London: Oxford University Press.
Horton, R. (2011) editorial, 'The making of a modern medic', *The Lancet* Vol. 377, May 28, p1807.

Hughes, J. C. (2006) 'Patterns of practice: a useful notion in medical ethics?' *Journal of Ethics in Mental Health* 1: 1–5.

—. (2011) *Thinking Through Dementia*. Oxford: Oxford University Press.

Hughes, J. C., Louw, S., and Sabat, S. (eds) (2006) *Dementia: Mind, Meaning and the Person*. Oxford/New York: Oxford University Press.

Hume, D. (1911) *A Treatise of Human Nature*. London: J. M. Dent and Sons.

Humphreys, C. (2000) *Undying spirits. Religion, medicine and institutionalized care for the dying, 1878–1938*. Ph.D. thesis, University of Sheffield.

—. (2001) 'Waiting for the last summons. The establishment of the first hospices in England 1878–1914'. *Mortality* 6(2): 146–166.

Husserl, E. (1977) *Cartesian Meditations: An Introduction to Phenomenology*. Cairns, D. (tr.). Dordrecht: Kluwer.

Huxtable, R. (2000) 'The court of appeal and conjoined twins: condemning the unworthy life?' *Bulletin of Medical Ethics* 162: 13–18.

—. (2007) *Euthanasia, Ethics and the Law: From Conflict to Compromise*. London: Routledge-Cavendish.

—. (2010) 'Calculating the value of life?' In: Dickenson, D., Huxtable, R., and Parker, M. (ed.) *The Cambridge Medical Ethics Workbook* (2nd edn). Cambridge: Cambridge University Press, pp. 2–3.

Huxtable, R. and Moller, M. (2007) "Setting a principled boundary'? Euthanasia as a response to 'life fatigue". *Bioethics* 21(3): 117–126.

Illich, I. (2002) *Limits to Medicine: Medical Nemesis: The Expropriation of Health*. New York: Marion-Boyars.

Inwood, M. (1997) *Heidegger: A Very Short Introduction*. Oxford: Oxford University Press.

Irish Medical Council. (2009) *Guide to Professional Conduct and Ethics for Registered Medical Practitioners* (7th edn). Dublin: Irish Medical Council.

Jackson, L. and Huxtable, R. (2005) 'The doctor-parent relationship: as fragile as glass?' *Journal of Social Welfare and Family Law* 27(3–4): 369–381.

Jacobson, D. (2006) 'Seeing by feeling: virtues, skills, and moral perception'. *Ethical Theory and Moral Practice* 8(4): 387–409.

James, N. (1994) 'From vision to system. The maturing of the hospice movement'. In: Lee, R. and Morgan, D. (eds) *Death Rites*. London: Routledge, pp. 102–130.

Janssens, M. J. P. A. (1997) 'Lippendienst aan palliatieve zorg' [Lip service to palliative care]. *Trouw*, 28 March 1997.

Janssens, M. J. P. A., *et al.* (1999) 'Articulating the concept of palliative care. Philosophical and theological perspectives'. *Journal of Palliative Care* 15(2): 38–44.

—. (2002) 'Moral values in palliative care. A European comparison'. In: Ten Have, H. and Clark, D. (eds) *The Ethics of Palliative Care. European Perspectives*. Oxford: Oxford University Press, pp. 72–86.

Johnson, M. E. (1998) 'Being mentally ill: a phenomenological inquiry'. *Archives of Psychiatric Nursing* 12(4): 195–201.

Jonas, H. (1992/1979) *The Imperative of Responsibility. In Search of an Ethics for the Technological Age*. Jonas, H. and Herr, D. (trs.). Chicago-London: The University of Chicago Press.

Jones, D. A. (2006) 'The Hippocratic Oath II: modern adaptations of the classical doctors' oath'. *Catholic Medical Quarterly* 56(1): 6–16.

Kaldjian, L. C., Jekel, J. F. and Friedland, G. (1998) 'End-of-life decisions in HIV-positive patients: the role of spiritual beliefs'. *AIDS* 12(1): 103–107.
Kant, I. (1998/1785) *Groundwork of the Metaphysics of Morals*. Gregor, M. J. (tr.). Cambridge: Cambridge University Press.
Katerndahl, D. A. (2008) 'Impact of spiritual symptoms and their interactions on health services and life satisfaction'. *Annals of Family Medicine* 6(5): 412–420.
Kearney, R. (2008) 'Vers une herméneutique de la traduction'. In: Fiasse, G. (ed.) *Paul Ricœur. De l'homme faillible à l'homme capable*. Paris: Presses universitaires de France, pp. 155–178.
Khushf, G. (ed.) (2004) *Handbook of Bioethics: Taking Stock of the Field from a Philosophical Perspective*. Dordrecht: Kluwer.
Killmister, S. (2010) 'Dignity: not such a useless concept'. *Journal of Medical Ethics* 36: 160–164.
Kitwood, T. (1997) *Dementia Reconsidered*. Buckingham/Philadelphia: Open University Press.
Koenig, H. G. (2008) *Medicine, Religion, and Health: Where Science and Spirituality Meet West*. Conshohocken, PA: Templeton Foundation Press.
Kübler-Ross, E. (1969) *On Death and Dying*. London: Tavistock.
Kuhse, H. and Singer, P. (eds) (2009) *A Companion to Bioethics* (2nd edn). Oxford: Wiley-Blackwell.
LaFollette, E. and LaFollette, H. (2007) 'Private conscience, public acts'. *Journal of Medical Ethics* 33: 249–254.
Lammers, A. and Cunningham, A. (eds) (2007) *The Jung-White Letters*. London: Routledge.
Leder, D. (1990) *The Absent Body*. Chicago, IL: The University of Chicago Press.
Levin, A. (2009) '80 lawyers refused to help save Baby OT, leaving the parents to fend for themselves'. *The Daily Mail*, 22 March 2009.
Levin, J. S. (1994) 'Religion and health: is there an association, is it valid, and is it causal?' *Social Science & Medicine* 38(11): 1475–1482.
Levitt, M. (2003) 'Public consultation in bioethics. What's the point of asking the public when they have neither scientific nor ethical expertise?' *Health Care Analysis* 11(1): 15–25.
Lewis, M. (2005) *Heidegger and the Place of Ethics*. London: Continuum.
Low, L., King, S. and Wilkie, T. (1998) 'Genetic discrimination in life insurance: empirical evidence from a cross sectional survey of genetic support groups in the United Kingdom'. *British Medical Journal* 317: 1632–1635.
Lucassen, A. and Parker, M. (2004) 'Confidentiality and serious harm in genetics—preserving the confidentiality of one patient and preventing harm to relatives'. *European Journal of Human Genetics* 12: 93–97.
Luntley, M. (2003) *Wittgenstein: Meaning and Judgement*. Malden USA/Oxford/Carlton Australia: Blackwell.
MacIntyre, A. (1999) *Dependent Rational Animals*. London: Duckworth and Co. Ltd.
—. (2007) *After Virtue* (1981/1997/2007) *After Virtue* (1st, 2nd, 3rd eds). Notre Dame: University of Notre Dame Press..
Mack, E. (1989) 'Dominos and the fear of commodification'. In: Chapman, J. W. and Pennock, J. R. (eds) *Markets and Justice, Nomos XXXI*. New York: New York University Press.

Maclean, A. (1993) *The Elimination of Morality: Reflections on Utilitarianism and Bioethics.* London: Routledge.

Malmqvist, E. and Zeiler, K. (2010) 'Cultural norms, the phenomenology of incorporation and the experience of having a child born with ambiguous sex'. *Social Theory and Practice* 36(1): 157–164.

May, T. (2002) *Bioethics in a Liberal Society. The Political Framework of Bioethics Decision Making.* Baltimore, MD: Johns Hopkins UP.

May, W. F. (1975) 'Code, covenant, contract, or philanthropy'. *The Hastings Center Report* 5(6): 29–38.

McLean, S. A. M. (2007a) 'Law, ethics and health care'. In: Ashcroft, R. E., Dawson, A. Draper, H. and McMillan, J. R. (eds) *Principles of Health Care Ethics* (2nd edn). Chichester: John Wiley and Sons, pp. 193–198.

—. (2007b) 'What and who are clinical ethics committees for?' *Journal of Medical Ethics* 33: 497–500.

—. (2008) 'Clinical ethics committees: a due process wasteland?' *Clinical Ethics* 3: 99–104.

Merchant, R., *et al.* (2007) 'Patients' emergency contraception comprehension, usage, and view of the emergency department role for emergency contraception'. *The Journal of Emergency Medicine* 33(4): 367–375.

Merleau-Ponty, M. (2006/1945) *Phenomenology of Perception.* Smith, C. (tr.). London: Routledge and Kegan Paul.

Mill, J. S. (1985/1859) *On Liberty.* London: Penguin.

Miller, P. S. (2000) 'Is there a pink slip in my genes? Genetic discrimination in the workplace'. *Journal of Health Care Law and Policy* 3: 225–265.

Miyasaki, D. (2007) 'A ground for ethics in Heidegger's being and time'. *Journal of the British Society for Phenomenology* 38(3): 261–279.

Moran, D. (2000) *Introduction to Phenomenology.* London: Routledge.

Moran, G. (2005) 'Maternal wish, doctors' faith at odds in court'. *The San Diego Union-Tribune,* 7 August 2005, p. A1.

Morrison, W. (1997) *Jurisprudence: From the Greeks to Post-Modernism.* London: Cavendish.

Neeleman, J., Halpern, D., Leon, D. and Lewis, G. (1997) 'Tolerance of suicide, religion and suicide rates: an ecological and individual study in 19 Western countries'. *Psychological Medicine* 27: 1165–1171.

Newman, J. H. (1990/1852) *The Idea of a University.* Notre Dame: University of Notre Dame Press.

Nozick, R. (1974) *Anarchy, State and Utopia.* Oxford: Blackwell.

Nuffield Council on Bioethics. (2006) *Critical Care Decisions in Fetal and Neonatal Medicine: Ethical Issues.* London: Nuffield Council on Bioethics.

Nussbaum, M. (1990) *Love's Knowledge: Essays on Philosophy and Literature.* Oxford/New York: Oxford University Press.

—. (1999) 'Virtue ethics: a misleading category?' *Journal of Ethics* 3(3): 163–201.

O'Donoghue, J. (2009) *Sectioned: A Life Interrupted.* London: John Murray.

O'Neill, O. (2002) *Autonomy and Trust in Bioethics.* Cambridge: Cambridge University Press.

Oderberg, D. S. (2000) *Applied Ethics: A Non-Consequentialist Approach.* Oxford: Blackwell Publishers.

Orr, R. D. and Genesen, L. B. (1997) 'Requests for "inappropriate" treatment based on religious beliefs'. *Journal Medical Ethics* 23: 142–147.

Paley, W. (2006/1802) *Natural Theology*. Oxford: Oxford University Press.

Parfit, D. (1984) *Reasons and Persons*. Oxford: Clarendon Press.

Parsons, E. and Atkinson, P. (1992) 'Lay constructions of genetic risk'. *Sociology of Health and Illness* 14(4): 437–455.

Pearson, G. and Salter, M. (1999) 'Getting public law back into a critical condition: the rule of law as a source for immanent critique'. *Social and Legal Studies* 8(4): 483–508.

Pellegrino, E. D. (1993) *The Virtues in Medical Practice*. New York: Oxford University Press.

—. (1995) 'Toward a virtue-based normative ethics for the health professions'. *Kennedy Institute of Ethics Journal* 5(3): 253–277.

—. (2001) 'The internal morality of clinical medicine: a paradigm for the ethics of the helping and healing profession'. *Journal of Medicine and Philosophy* 26(6): 559–579.

—. (2002) 'The physician's conscience, conscience clauses, and religious beliefs: a Catholic perspective'. *Fordham Urban Law Journal* 30: 221–244.

Pellegrino, E. D. and Thomasma, D. (1981) *A Philosophical Basis of Medical Practice: Toward a Philosophy and Ethic of the Healing Professions*. New York: Oxford University Press.

Phillips, J. (2004) 'Psychopathology and the narrative self'. *Philosophy, Psychiatry & Psychology* 10(4): 313–328

Pieranunzi, V. R. (1997) 'The lived expeirence of power and powerlessness in psychiatric nursing: a Heideggerian hermeneutical analysis'. *Archives of Psychiatric Nursing* 11(3): 155–162.

Pierron, J.-P. (2010) *Vulnérabilité. Pour une philosophie du soin*. Paris: Presses universitaires de France.

Polanyi, M. (1958) *Personal Knowledge. Towards a Post-Critical Philosophy*. London: Routledge & Kegan Paul.

Pritchard, D. (2005) *Epistemic Luck*. Oxford: Clarendon Press.

Qualtere-Burcher, P. (2009) 'The just distance: narrativity, singularity, and relationality as the source of a new biomedical principle'. *The Journal of Clinical Ethics* 20: 299–309.

Radcliffe-Richards, J., Daar, A. S., Guttmann, R. D., Hoffenberg, R., Kennedy, I., Lock, M., Sells, R. A. and Tilney, N. (1998) 'The case for allowing kidney sales. International forum for transplant ethics'. *The Lancet* 351: 1950–1952.

Radin, M. J. (1996) *Contested Commodities*. Cambridge, MA: Harvard University Press.

—. (1989) 'Reconsidering the rule of law'. *Boston University Law Review* 69(4): 781–819.

Rai, G. (ed.) (2004) *Medical Ethics and the Elderly* (2nd edn). Oxford/San Francisco: Radcliffe Medical Press.

Räikkä, J. (1998) 'Freedom and a right (not) to know'. *Bioethics* 12(1): 49–63.

Ratcliffe, M. (2009) 'Understanding existential changes in psychiatric illness: the indispensability of phenomenology'. In: Broome, M. and Bortolotti, L. (eds) *Psychiatry as Cognitive Neuroscience*. Oxford: Oxford University Press, pp. 223–244.

Ravnskov, U., Rosch, P. J., Sutter, M. C. and Houston, M. C. (2006) 'Should we lower cholesterol as much as possible?' *British Medical Journal* 332: 1330–1332.

Rawls, J. (1972) *A Theory of Justice*. Oxford: Oxford University Press.

Raz, J. (1977) 'The rule of law and its virtue'. *The Law Quarterly Review* 93: 195–211.

Rees, C. and Monrouxe, L. V. (2011) 'Medical students learning intimate examinations without valid consent: a multicentre study,'. *Medical Education* 45: 261–271.

Rees, P. (2009a) 'Harlequins fined and Tom Williams suspended in fake blood injury case'. *The Guardian*, 20 July 2009.

—. (2009b) 'Former Harlequins physio Steph Brennan struck off over Bloodgate'. *The Guardian*, 14 September 2009.

Rehmann-Sutter, C., Düwell, M., *et al.* (eds) (2006) *Bioethics in Cultural Contexts. Reflections on Methods and Finitude*. Dordrecht: Springer.

Rescher, N. (1983) *Risk: A Philosophical Introduction*. Washington, DC: University Press of America.

—. (1993) 'Moral luck'. In: Statman, D. (ed.) *Moral Luck*. Albany, NY: SUNY Press, pp. 141–166.

—. (1995) *Luck*. Pittsburg: Pittsburg University Press.

Rhodes, R. (1998) 'Genetic links, family ties, and social bonds: rights and responsibilities in the face of genetic knowledge'. *Journal of Medicine and Philosophy* 23(1): 10–30.

—. (2000) 'Autonomy, respect and genetic information policy: a reply to Tuija Takala and Matti Häyry'. *Journal of Medicine and Philosophy* 25(1): 114–120.

—. (2006) 'The ethical standard of care'. *American Journal of Bioethics* 6(2): 76–78.

Richards, M. (2001) 'How distinctive is genetic information?' *Studies in History and Philosophy of Biological and Biomedical Sciences* 32(4): 663–687.

Richards, M. and Ponder, M. (1996) 'Lay understanding of genetics: a test of a hypothesis'. *Journal of Medical Genetics* 33: 1032–1036.

Richardson, R. (1987) *Death, Dissection, and the Destitute*. London/New York: Routledge and Kegan Paul.

Richmond, C. (2005) 'Dame Cicely Saunders'. *British Medical Journal* 331(7510): 238.

Ricœur, P. (1992a) *Oneself as Another*. Blamey, K. (tr.). Chicago, IL: The University of Chicago Press.

—. (1992b) 'La souffrance n'est pas la douleur'. *Psychiatrie française* numéro spécial 92: 9–18.

—. (1993) 'Responsibility and fragility: an ethical reflection'. *The Journal of the Faculty of Religious Studies (McGill University)* 21: 7–10.

—. (1996) 'Préface'. In: *Code de déontologie médicale*, Introd. et commenté par L. René. Paris: Seuil.

—. (2000a) 'Prudential judgement, deontological judgement and reflexive judgement in medical ethics'. In: Kemp, P. and Rendtorff, J. *et al.* (eds) *Bioethics and Biolaw. Vol. I: Judgement of Life*. Copenhagen: Rhodos International Science and Art Publishers & Centre for Ethics and Law.

—. (2000b) *The Just*. Pellauer, D. (tr.). Chicago, IL: The University of Chicago Press.

—. (2001) 'The just and medical ethics'. In: Thomasma, D. C. (ed.) *Personhood and Health Care*. Dordrecht: Kluwer Academic Publishers, pp. 115–119.

—. (2002) 'Ethics and human capability. A response'. In: Wall, J. and Schweiker, W. (eds) *Paul Ricœur and Contemporary Moral Thought*. New York: Routledge, pp. 279–290.

—. (2005) *The Course of Recognition*. Pellauer, D. (tr.). Cambridge, MA: Harvard University Press.
—. (2006) *On Translation*. Brennan, E. (tr.). New York: Routledge.
—. (2007a) *Reflections on the Just*. Pellauer, D. (tr.). Chicago, IL: The University of Chicago Press.
—. (2007b) 'From the moral to the ethical and to ethics'. Ricœur 2007a, pp. 45–57.
—. (2007c) 'Autonomy and vulnerability'. Ricœur 2007a, pp. 72–90.
—. (2007d) 'The Paradigm of translation'. Ricœur 2007a, pp. 106–122.
—. (2007e) 'The difference between the normal and the pathological as a source of respect'. Ricœur 2007a, pp. 187–197.
—. (2007f) 'The three levels of medical judgment'. Ricœur 2007a, pp. 198–212.
—. (2007g) 'Decision making in medical and judicial judgments'. Ricœur 2007a, pp. 213–222.
—. (2010) 'Asserting personal capacities and pleading for mutual recognition'. In: Treanor, B. and Venema, H. I. (eds) *A Passion for the Possible. Thinking with Paul Ricœur*. New York: Fordham UP, pp. 22–26.
Risse, G. B. (1999) *Mending Bodies, Saving Souls: A History of Hospitals*. Oxford: Oxford University Press.
Romdenh-Romluc, K. (2011) *The Routledge Guidebook to Merleau-Ponty and Phenomenology of Perception*. Abingdon/New York: Routledge.
Ross, A. and Athanassoulis, N. (2011) 'Virtue ethics and risk'. In: Roeser, S. (ed.) *The Handbook of Risk Theory*. Amsterdam: Springer.
Roy, D., *et al.* (1994) 'Regarding euthanasia'. *European Journal for Palliative Care* 1(1): 57–59.
Royal Liverpool Children's Inquiry. (2001) *Report of the Royal Liverpool Children's Inquiry*. London: Stationery Office.
Ryle, G. (1949) *The Concept of Mind*. London: Hutchinson.
Sadler, J. Z. (2004) *Values and Psychiatric Diagnosis*. Oxford: Oxford University Press.
Saunders, C. (1960a) 'Drug treatment in the terminal stages of cancer'. *Current Medicine and Drugs* 1(1): 16–28.
—. (1960b) 'Care of the dying'. *Nursing Times Supplement* 72(26): 1003–1005.
—. (1965a) 'Telling patients'. *District Nursing*, September 1965, pp. 149–154.
—. (1965b) 'The last stages of life'. *American Journal of Nursing* 65: 70–75.
—. (1966) 'The management of terminal illness'. *British Journal of Hospital Medicine* (December), 225–228.
—. (1995) 'Preface'. In: Saunders, C., *et al. Living with Dying. A Guide to Palliative Care*. Oxford: Oxford University Press.
Savulescu, J. (2006) 'Conscientious objection in medicine'. *British Medical Journal* 332: 294–297.
Secular Medical Forum. (2009) Accessed March 2011, www.secularmedicalforum.org.uk.
Sidgwick, H. (1891) *The Elements of Politics*. London: Macmillan.
Sinclair, S. (1997) *Making Doctors: An Institutional Apprenticeship*. Oxford/New York: Berg.
Singer, P. and Viens, A. (eds) (2008) *The Cambridge Textbook of Bioethics*. Cambridge: Cambridge University Press.

Sitvast, J. E., Abma, T. A., *et al.* (2008) 'Photo stories, Ricœur, and experiences from practice. A hermeneutic dialogue'. *Advances in Nursing Science* 31: 268–279.

Skene, L. (1998) 'Patients' rights or family responsibilities? Two approaches to genetic testing'. *Medical Law Review* 6: 1–41.

Sloan, R. P., Bagiella, E., VandeCreek, L., *et al.* (2000) 'Should physicians prescribe religious activities?' *New England Journal of Medicine* 342: 1913–1916.

Smart, J. J. C. and Williams, B. (1973) *Utilitarianism: For and Against.* Cambridge: Cambridge University Press.

Steinbock, B. (ed.) (2009) *The Oxford Handbook of Bioethics.* Oxford: Oxford University Press.

Stichter, M. (2007) 'Ethical expertise: the skill model of virtue'. *Ethical Theory and Moral Practice* 10(2): 183–194.

Sugarman, J. and Sulmasy, D. P. (eds) (2001) *Methods in Medical Ethics.* Washington, DC: Georgetown University Press.

Sulmasy, D. (2008) 'What is conscience and why is respect for it so important?' *Theoretical Medicine and Bioethics* 29: 135–149.

Sykora, P. (2010) 'Altruism in medical donations reconsidered: the reciprocity approach'. In: Steinmann, M., Sykora, P., and Wiesing, U. (eds) *Altruism Reconsidered: Exploring New Approaches to Property in Human Tissue.* Aldershot: Ashgate.

Szasz, T. and Hollender, M. H. (1956) 'A contribution to the philosophy of medicine: the basic models of the doctor-patient relationship'. *Archives of Internal Medicine* 97: 585–592.

Taiëb, O., Révah-Lévy, A., *et al.* (2008) 'Is Ricœur's notion of narrative identity useful in understanding recovery in drug addicts?' *Qualitative Health Research* 18: 990–1000.

Taiëb, O., Reyre, A., *et al.*(2010) 'La promesse dans les addictions: de la reconnaissance de soi à la reconnaissance mutuelle selon Hannah Arendt et Paul Ricœur'. *Psychotropes* 16: 21–34.

Takala, T. (1999) 'The right to genetic ignorance confirmed'. *Bioethics* 13(3/4): 288–293.

Takala, T. and Häyry, M. (2000) 'Genetic ignorance, moral obligations and social duties'. *Journal of Medicine and Philosophy* 25(1): 107–113.

Taylor, C. (1991) *The Ethics of Authenticity.* Cambridge, MA: Harvard University Press.

Thomasma, D. (2000) *The Health Care Professional as a Friend and Healer.* Washington, DC: Georgetown University Press.

Thornton, T. (2007) *Essential Philosophy of Psychiatry.* Oxford: Oxford University Press.

Titmuss, R. M. (1970) *The Gift Relationship: From Human Blood to Social Policy.* London: George Allen and Unwin.

Tolstoy, L. N. (1998/1886) *The Death of Ivan Ilych.* The Pennsylvania State University, Electronic Classics Series. Accessed April 2011, available at: http://www.scribd.com/doc/7108120/The-Death-of-Ivan-Ilych-by-Leo-Tolstoy.

Tong, R. (1998) 'The ethics of care: a feminist virtue ethics of care for healthcare practitioners'. *Journal of Medicine and Philosophy* 23(2): 131–152.

Tottenham, M. (1995) 'Case comment on medical council: fitness to practice—report of fitness to practice committee'. *Medico-Legal Journal of Ireland* 14: 16–19.

Trost, J. (1990) 'Do we mean the same by the concept of family?' *Communication Research* 17: 431–443.

Twining, W. and Miers, D. R. (1991) *How to Do Things with Rules* (3rd edn). London: Butterworths.

Van Dam, H. (1997) 'Palliatieve zorg en euthanasie. Valse tegenstellingen' [Palliative care and euthanasia. False contradictions]. *Trouw*, 4 April, 1997.

Waltz, E. (2006) 'The body snatchers'. *Nature Medicine* 12: 487–488.

Ward Platt, M. and Ward Platt, A. (2005) 'Conflicts of care'. *Archives of Disease in Childhood* 90(4): 331.

Warnock, M. and Macdonald, E. (2008) *Easeful Death; Is There a Case for Assisted Dying?* Oxford: Oxford University Press.

Weber, M. (1968) *Economy and Society: An Outline of Interpretive Sociology*. Roth, G. and Wittich, C. (eds) Fischoff, E., *et al.* (trs.). New York: Bedminster Press.

Weldon, C. (2007) *Fr. Victor White, O. P.: the story of Jung's 'White Raven'*. Scranton, PA: University of Scranton Press.

White, A. D. (1896) *The Warfare of Science with Theology in Christendom Volume II*. New York: D Appleton & Company. Accessed March 2011, <http://www.general-anaesthesia.com/science-theology/index.html>.

White, V. (1960) *Soul and Psyche*. London, Collins and Harvill Press.

WHO. (2002) *National Cancer Control Programmes: Policies and Managerial Guidelines*. Geneva: World Health Organization.

Wicclair, M. R. (1993) *Ethics and the Elderly*. New York/Oxford: Oxford University Press.

—. (2008) 'Is conscientious objection incompatible with a physician's professional obligations?' *Theoretical Medicine and Bioethics* 29(3): 171–185.

—. (2011) *Conscientious Objection in Health Care: An Ethical Analysis*. Cambridge: Cambridge University Press.

Widdershoven, G. (2002) 'Beyond autonomy and beneficence: the moral basis of euthanasia in the Netherlands'. *Ethical Perspectives* 9(2): 96–102.

Widdershoven, G., *et al.* (2007) 'Hermeneutic ethics between practice and theory'. In: Ashcroft, R. E., *et al.* (eds) *Principles of Health Care Ethics*. London: Wiley and Sons.

—. (2009) 'Empirical ethics as dialogical practice'. *Bioethics* 23(4): 236–238.

Wilkinson, R. H. (2010a) 'When is my genetic information your business? Biological, emotional and financial claims to knowledge'. *Cambridge Quarterly of Healthcare Ethics* 19: 1–8.

—. (2010b) 'Unjustified discrimination: is the moratorium on the use of genetic information by insurers a contradiction in terms?' *Health Care Analysis* 18(3): 279–293.

Wilkinson, S. (2003) *Bodies for Sale: Ethics and Exploitation in the Human Body Trade*. London/New York: Routledge.

Williams, J. D. (1874) *History of the Conflict between Religion and Science*. New York: D Appleton.

Wittgenstein, L. (1969) *On Certainty*. Anscombe, G. E. M. and von Wright, G. H. (eds) Paul, D. and Anscombe, G. E. M. (trs.). Oxford: Blackwell.

—. (1981). *Zettel*. Anscombe, G. E. M. and von Wright, G. H. (eds) Anscombe, G. E. M. (tr.). Oxford: Blackwell.

Zeiler, K. (2012) 'A Phenomenology of Excorporation: Rethinking Embodiment and Agency', unpublished manuscript.

Zimmerman, M. (1993) 'Luck and moral responsibility'. In: Statman, D. (ed.) *Moral Luck*. Albany, NY: State University of New York Press, pp. 217–234.

Legal cases

Airedale NHS Trust v Bland [1993] 2 WLR 816.

Arthur [1981] 12 BMLR 1.

Bolton v Law Society [1994] 1 WLR 512, 519.

Brennan v Health Professions Council [2011] EWHC 41.

An NHS Trust v MB [2006] EWHC 507.

Portsmouth Hospitals NHS Trust v Wyatt (Costs) [2006] EWCA Civ 529.

Portsmouth NHS Trust (No. 1) v Wyatt [2005a] EWHC 117.

Portsmouth NHS Trust v W [2005b] EWHC 2293.

Portsmouth NHS Trust v Wyatt [2004] 1 FLR 21.

Prendiville & Anor v Medical Council [2008] 3 IR 131

R v Portsmouth Hospitals NHS Trust ex p. Glass [1999] 2 FLR 905.

Re A (children) (conjoined twins: surgical separation) [2000] 4 All ER 961.

Re B (a minor) (wardship: medical treatment) [1981] 1 WLR 1421.

Re C (Medical Treatment) [1998] 1 FLR 384.

Re Wyatt (A Child) (Medical Treatment: Continuation of Order) [2005] EWHC 693.

Re Wyatt [2006] EWHC 319.

Wyatt v Portsmouth Hospital NHS Trust [2005] EWCA Civ 1181.

Index